PRAISE FOR DIANA FRIEL McGOWIN AND *LIVING IN THE LABYRINTH,* AN INTIMATE ACCOUNT OF ONE WOMAN'S BATTLE WITH ALZHEIMER'S

"McGowin writes bluntly about coping with the disease . . . about being angry with friends who didn't understand . . . and about her frustrations. Her purpose is to tell victims that they aren't alone." —*The Miami Herald*

"McGowin's brilliant, thoroughly engrossing narrative is for victims, professionals, friends, family, and those of us who want to walk for a few hours in the shoes of . . . an Alzheimer's victim." —*Health & Fitness*

"A unique and valuable source of insight into the inner world and feelings of the person with A.D. Intimate and deeply moving." —Carmel Sheridan, author of *Failure-Free Activities for the Alzheimer's Patient*

"An excellent guide for professionals, friends and family . . . will bring light into the lives of other early-onset Alzheimer victims." —Mary Ellen Ort-Marvin, Board Member, Greater Orlando Alzheimer Association

"[*Living in the Labyrinth*] documents the plight of millions of us who live partially in the shadows because they are afflicted with A.D." —Dr. Richard Badessa, Professor Emeritus, University of Louisville (Alzheimer's victim)

"Outstanding. Must reading for patient and families. Should be read by all clergymen, physicians and counselors who deal with this difficult disease." —Dr. Thomas Dow, Orlando Professional Group

LIVING IN THE LABYRINTH

A Personal Journey Through The Maze Of Alzheimer's.

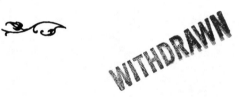

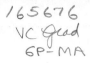

Diana Friel McGowin

Delta
Trade Paperbacks

In memory of my mother, Geneva Parrett Friel.

*This book is also dedicated to my bon homme
Richard,
Dr. Richard Badessa,
and all fellow travellers
on our journey through the labyrinth.
Thank you for walking with me.*

TABLE OF CONTENTS

Chapters

FOREWORD

*A*lzheimer's disease is well publicized today and books which describe the impact of the disease from the family and professional's standpoint are plentiful. While these are invaluable, their perspective is that of the caregiver, not the patient.

Living In The Labyrinth is unique in that it focuses on Alzheimer's disease from the patient's perspective. It is the gripping personal story of Diana Friel McGowin's struggle to gain control of her life while in the throes of the disease. While still in her forties, McGowin began to realize that her world was slipping away. Her book—the first so far to address the subject of early-onset Alzheimer's—takes us step by step from the first innocuous symptoms of confusion through the progressive stages of disability.

McGowin shows us that Alzheimer's disease is not a death sentence. Most people live for many years after being diagnosed, and the progression of the disease is individual and often gradual. As the author points out, there are plateaus in Alzheimer's, periods of time when losses level off and the condition stabilizes. Diana has been at a plateau for two years, and her condition may stabilize at this point for many years.

This is not a "poor me" chronicle; Diana's story is one of hope and like her, many patients can develop coping mechanisms which will help them get on with their lives. She shows that people can continue to enjoy their family, friends and former interests in spite of the limitations of Alzheimer's. Her message to caregivers is the profound need for love, understanding and support of the patient at each phase of the illness.

Living In The Labyrinth is a landmark book and the missing link in the literature on Alzheimer's.

Carmel Sheridan, M.A.
Author, **Failure-Free Activities for the Alzheimer's Patient**

ACKNOWLEDGMENTS

I am most deeply touched and appreciative of each and every act of friendship or kindness freely given to me by all my family, and most especially my friends from my past who, upon reuniting with me today, accept me with open and deep affection.

Particular thanks from my heart and soul I extend to my father for giving me the genetic backbone I needed to bring this to fruition; to my husband for attempting to change and supporting me; to Shaun, for his great wit, rapport and protectiveness; to Lynn and Steve, for always being there; to Bill and his wife, Julie, for kind Christian family concern; and to Jereme and Steven, for just being mine.

This book would not have been possible except for the kindness and supportive friendship/sisterhood of Mary Lou Sprowle and the initial inspiration by Kenneth Fulton.

I also express appreciation to Robert Thornton, M.D., Thomas Dow, M.D., and Mrs. Phyllis Dow, L.C.S.W., for their humane, concerned professionalism, and to Mary Ellen Ort-Marvin and other members of the local Board of the Alzheimer's Association for being there as I strive to maintain balance.

I embrace you all, tenderly.

INTRODUCTION

*W*hen I first received my diagnosis of Alzheimer's disease, I closed myself up in one room of my darkened and tightly locked house, and refused to answer the telephone or door bell. Although I had tried for years to determine what was happening to me, I was not prepared for the truth I was so frantically seeking.

You see, I had gone searching for something "fixable." Alzheimer's disease is not fixable. At present, it is considered terminal.

This book is a chronicle of my battle with Alzheimer's. It is a plain-language, "as it happened" chronicle which I pray will assist others like me who are dealing with this perplexing problem, and their families. It is a factual account of an average American family with nothing more than life's typical problems, until it experienced the confusion, anxiety and heartbreak of an unknown affliction. It catalogues the innocent mistakes made and the successful positive steps taken by a family with no rule book to refer to in coping with an often difficult and tragic situation.

I hope that it offers comfort to patients and their families and demonstrates that dignity is imperative for the survival of the self. The Alzheimer's patient asks nothing more than a hand to hold, a heart to care, and a mind to think for them when they cannot; someone to protect them as they travel through the dangerous twists and turns of the labyrinth.

These thoughts must be put on paper now. Tomorrow they may be gone, as fleeting as the bloom of night jasmine beside my front door.

Diana Friel McGowin
Orlando, Florida, 1992.

LIVING IN THE LABYRINTH

*A Personal Journey
Through The Maze
Of Alzheimer's.*

UNPLANNED JOURNEY

I hurried to put the finishing touches to the buffet table as the dining room clock chimed its warning cadence. My newly wed daughter, Lynn, and her husband, Lee, had arrived earlier for a visit, and I had invited the rest of my family for a small reunion and buffet luncheon.

Nervously, I checked off the table appointments on a list retrieved from my jumpsuit pocket. Such a list had never been necessary before, but lately I noticed frequent little episodes of confusion and memory lapses. It was probably tension, due to my hectic career. If it worsened, I would make an appointment for a checkup, to ensure that my previous difficulties with hypertension had not risen from the dead. I was proud of the fact that with dietary changes and exercise, my blood pressure problems had abated. A small stroke a couple of years ago, which my doctor had called a "transient ischemic attack," or TIA, had served as a warning to make these modest lifestyle changes.

Everything was on the table to my satisfaction. I took my purse from the kitchen shelf and hastened out the door to my car. It was now time to pick up the food from the restaurant nearby. I had decided to "cheat" on this family buffet, and have the meal prepared on a carry-out basis. Cooking was also becoming increasingly difficult, due to what my children and my husband Jack teasingly referred to as my "absentmindedness."

I returned home and carried in the food trays just as my son Bill, my brother, and their families arrived. Immediately thereafter my father arrived with my stepmother, and the pandemonium of chattering voices, the running feet of little children, and general family get-together noisiness began.

As darkness fell, we were all assembled on the patio deck. Large floodlights illuminated the backyard, and Polynesian torches were strategically placed around the deck. This practice delighted the children, as always.

Bill, together with Lynn and the youngest of the brood, Shaun, were still playfully recording the events of the day with a video camcorder. Lynn called out to me for another blank tape cassette, and I rushed inside to get one.

As I returned to the deck, I suddenly staggered, as the wooden deck appeared to heave and quake before me. I caught my balance by throwing myself against the exterior wall of the house.

"Okay, Sis! No more cola drinks for you!" my brother jested.

"What's the matter, Mom? Did your heel catch in the planking of the deck?" Lynn asked.

I knew God had given me this child for some reason! Shaken, I smiled in agreement and handed Lynn the blank cassette. The rest of the evening went without a hitch, as my kith and kin enjoyed exchanging familiarities and jokes while finishing off the food trays.

After our visitors left and Lynn and her husband retired to the guest room, Jack and I began the cleanup. My family had ravenously eaten everything but the paper plates, bones, and a few pieces of garlic bread. I smiled to myself in satisfaction, certain that they had all had a great time.

As Jack and I were sinking gratefully into bed, he questioned me about the "dizzy spell" on the deck.

"It wasn't a dizzy spell," I sighed. "I just lost my footing for a minute."

"I've noticed you having a lot of little 'losses' lately. When are you due for your next physical?"

I turned my back to him, not answering. That was the third time that day that I had momentarily lost my balance, although I did not feel faint or dizzy. It was as though someone was suddenly moving the earth beneath my feet, causing me to stagger or trip.

Jack advised me to telephone my doctor the next day and arrange for an examination, "just to be on the safe side."

The next morning, Lynn and her husband packed

their sedan immediately after breakfast. They wanted to be on the road early and avoid Florida's heat as they returned to their Tennessee home.

I fought tears as the young couple drove from the driveway. I missed the days when all the children were at home. Shaun would also be leaving in a few years. Even now, his life was so full with schooling and a busy social scene that he was rarely home.

I chided myself for too-early symptoms of empty nest syndrome. It was that time of life. My battle with little memory losses and balance were probably all psychosomatic, just a woman realizing that she was getting older, and not necessarily better. After all, I was forty-five years of age. One would naturally expect some innocuous symptoms of the body slowing down.

I set about catching up on household chores, but the family get-together had fatigued me. Opening a soft drink, I sank into my favorite easy chair, grateful to have the rest of the week off work.

Shaun walked past me on his way to the kitchen, and paused.

"Mom, what's up? You look ragged," he commented sleepily.

"Late night last night, plenty of excitement, and then up early to get your father off to work," I answered.

Shaun laughed disconcertingly.

I glanced up at him ruefully. "What is so funny?" I demanded.

"You, Mom! You are talking as though you are on a drunk or something! You must really be tired!"

The telephone rang, preventing a further retort from me. It was my husband, asking me to prepare a lunch and deliver it to him at his work-place. He would only have a thirty-minute lunch break; not enough time to get to a restaurant.

Quickly I put together a rudimentary lunch, and went to my car. I hesitated for a moment, confused on exactly how to place both my purse and the lunch container on the seat beside me. After some juggling, I backed the car from the driveway.

As I drove to Jack's office, I noticed a strip shopping center, new to me. It was strange I had not noticed this mall previously. I traveled this route frequently.

I passed the street leading to the off-site, and drove several miles down the road before realizing my error. No doubt the new shopping center had thrown my judgment off, I mused, and turned around to retrace my steps.
Near the driveway leading to my husband's office, I observed a fire station which was also new to me. That would be a good landmark to guide me to the company entrance in the future.

Jack saw my car approaching and came out of his building to greet me. Accepting the lunch with thanks, he leaned against the car.

"Jack, when did they build that new strip shopping center on Kirkman Road? Funny, but I don't remember it being built, and it is already open for business."

Jack frowned thoughtfully, then shook his head. I continued, "Oh, well, I'm glad to see the new fire station near your entrance. It will give me a good landmark."

Jack laughed and again shook his head.

"Diane, that station has always been here," he chided. "Even before my building was built!"

I suddenly became irate. I started the car and began to pull away from Jack, who leaped from his position leaning against the vehicle.

"Whoa! What's your rush?"

I braked, staring before me in confusion. Where was the exit?

"Jack," I asked shakily, "How do I get out of here?"

Jack now roared with laughter. "Diane, shape up! You certainly have something on your mind! 'New' shopping centers, 'new' fire stations, and now you can't find your way out of a parking lot!"

I fought tears of frustration as I shouted at Jack, "Don't laugh at me! Just tell me how to get out of this place!"

Jack bowed ceremoniously and pointed straight ahead of my car.

Without another word, I pulled away and drove from the parking lot.

Suddenly, I was aware of car horns blowing. Glancing around, nothing was familiar. I was stopped at an intersection and the traffic light was green. Cars honked impatiently, so I pulled straight ahead, trying to get my bearings. I could not read the street sign, but there was another sign ahead; perhaps it would shed some light on my location.

One of my favorite songs was playing on the radio. I was still in unfamiliar territory, at another intersection, in the right-hand turn lane. I took the turn, and spotted an overpass ahead. There were usually signs indicating the name of the roadway at overpasses. Now I could get my bearings.

The news was now coming over on the radio and I was alarmed to notice how fast I was driving. Where was the overpass? I looked around and discovered I was in open country, with a golf course to my left. Where was I? What was the matter with the radio? I slowed down to a safe speed, and read the name of the golf course on an entrance way. It was unfamiliar.

I drove on, with tears of frustration streaming down my face. Unfamiliar music blared from the radio. I could no longer see any buildings. I was hopelessly lost, and had no idea how to get home. Suddenly I saw a sign on a rock-walled entrance: "Turkey Lake Park." That struck a chord. Hadn't I taken the grandchildren to this park on several occasions?

I turned into the entrance of the park and pulled off the road. My body was shaking with fear and uncontrollable sobs. What was happening? An irritatingly boisterous commercial was playing on the radio. I snapped it off in annoyance and tried to clear my head.

A few yards ahead, there was a park ranger building. Trembling, I wiped my eyes, and breathing deeply, tried to calm myself. Finally, feeling ready to speak, I started the car again and approached the ranger station. The guard smiled and inquired how he could assist me.

"I appear to be lost," I began, making a great effort to keep my voice level, despite my emotional state.

"Where do you need to go?" the guard asked politely.

A cold chill enveloped me as I realized I could not remember the name of my street. Tears began to flow down my cheeks. I did not know where I wanted to go.

He prompted me, his voice soft as he noticed my tears.

"Are you heading to Orlando, or Windermere?"

"Orlando!" I sighed gratefully. That was right. I lived in Orlando. I was certain of it. But where?

"Which part? East end, West end?" the guard continued.

I felt panic wash over me anew as I searched my memory and found it blank. Suddenly, I remembered bringing my grandchildren to this park. That must mean I lived relatively nearby, surely.

"What is the closest subdivision?" I quavered.

The guard scratched his head thoughtfully.

"The closest Orlando subdivision would be Pine Hills, maybe," he ventured.

"That's right!" I exclaimed gratefully. The name of my subdivision had rung a bell.

The guard told me which way to turn as I left the park and to continue on that roadway until I approached the Colonial Avenue intersection. If I looked to my right, he instructed, I would see the entrance to the Pine Hills subdivision.

I drove carefully in the exact direction he advised and searched each intersection to see if it were Colonial Avenue. Finally, I came to it and looking to my right, recognized the entrance to the subdivision. I negotiated the streets leading to my home without further difficulty.

Once home, a wave of relief brought more tears. I rushed through my home, closing drapes and ensuring all doors were locked. I looked at my bedroom clock. I had been gone over four hours. I took refuge in the darkened master bedroom, and sat, curled up on my bed, my arms wrapped tightly around myself.

It was thus that Jack found me when he returned home that evening.

I would not at first answer Jack's queries as to why I was so depressed, but as he pressed, a torrent of tears spilled from me. I related all I could recall of the wretched day's events. Jack had no explanation, but only looked at me with a puzzled expression.

"I should have realized something was wrong when

you brought my lunch," he finally stated. "You weren't right, then. I thought you were preoccupied, or something."

The telephone rang with a call from Elise, my dearest friend for over twenty years. Jack briefly told Elise that I did not feel up to talking, and why. Elise was a nurse, and demanded that Jack put me on the telephone.

I tried to delineate the day's confusing pattern to Elise, but she soon interrupted and said she was coming over, immediately, and hung up.

Elise sat with me a long while, as I again attempted to sort out the day's events. I could not account for my whereabouts for four hours. It could not take that long to drive home from Jacks' office, even if one became lost for a while.

Jack interjected that he had checked the car's fuel gauge, and it appeared I had driven out an entire tank of gasoline that afternoon.

Elise insisted that I contact my neurologist immediately. I refused, stating I was afraid I "had lost my mind." Besides, I was home now, no emergency, and it was after hours.

Elise instructed Jack to see that I went to the neurologist's office first thing in the morning, and he agreed.

"Diane, if anything else occurs later tonight, call his emergency number immediately!"

At Jack's promise to follow her instructions, Elise departed. ✦

2

Initial Testing

I sat in the neurologist's office, then impatiently rose
to my feet and began pacing. This would probably
look strange to the receptionist, but who cared? I was
jittery with nerves, and still frightened that my mind
had "snapped," and I had become a basket case.

Finally, my neurologist appeared at the doorway, personally escorting me to his "inner sanctum," a walnut-
paneled and darkly furnished office. He sat behind
his enormous cluttered desk, and instructed me to sit
in the chair in front.

As I attempted to describe the reason for this visit, I
began crying. Chagrined, I gave up all hope of conducting myself in a professional manner, and
implored the neurologist to explain my dilemma.

"We must first run some tests, Diane," he stated crisply.
"Fortunately, we have the original results of the electroencephalogram, or EEG, which we conducted a few

11

years ago when you had a stroke. Isn't that correct?
Hmm, and we also performed a preliminary magnetic
resonance imagery, or MRI, at that time," he continued, leafing through my chart.

"First, let's step over to the examining room and see
how we're doing." He smiled. I loathed his habit of
referring to me in the first person plural, "we,"
"our," "us." I was tempted to ask him if he had a
mouse in his pocket. After he escorted me to another room equipped with the customary gurney
table and chrome fixtures, I obediently went through
the various examining procedures. He checked my
reflexes, instructed me to follow lights with my eyes,
walk a straight line, then stand on one leg with arms
outstretched. Finally, he requested me to count back-
wards from one hundred.

At the end of the examination, he stated that "we" had
performed all those tasks without any difficulty, and
now he was going to request another EEG and MRI, to
compare with my previous results. This would alleviate any suspicion of a brain tumor, and determine if I
had sustained another minor stroke.

I drove to the neurological testing facility and had no
difficulty finding a parking spot near the door. Inside,
the receptionist handed me a two-page form to complete, listing statistical information, insurance carrier,
and all medical history.

I had difficulty completing the portion of my own
medical history and asked the receptionist again if
they could look at the form I completed a few years
ago. She shook her head, stating she needed my new
form.

I returned to my seat, and made another attempt to remember the required information. Suddenly, in aggravated vehemence, I scribbled across the form, "If I could remember these details, I would not be here!" I held onto the form until the technician came to escort me to the testing room.

The technician attached my form to the chart of my previous visit, and instructed me to lie down on the padded vinyl examining table.

"Having a little difficulty with your memory?"

"A lot," I answered.

"When did this begin?"

"I don't remember," I laughed ruefully, then attempted to give a better answer. "I believe it has been just a few weeks, maybe more, maybe less, but the worst was yesterday. I lost four hours and drove out a tank full of gas. I was trying to drive home through very familiar territory."

"Any other problems?"

"I have had slight balance problems, not regularly, not very often, and not dizziness, just balance."

The technician explained the electroencephalogram (EEG) procedure, reminding me that I had undergone it a few years ago. The test began, and I was quite relaxed in the darkness. I kept my eyes closed while colored lights were flashed before my face. The lights were so bright that, even with my eyes closed, I could visualize vibrant flashes of color, pulsating in various rhythms. In a matter of minutes, the test was completed, and I was moved to another building for the magnetic resonance imaging (MRI) test.

The receptionist in that building also requested that I complete the medical history form. This time, however, I simply wrote across it neatly that I had no accurate recall of the requested information and to please refer to previous testing.

For the MRI procedure, I changed into a white hospital gown, and again lay upon a vinyl covered table. A large drum-shaped cylinder was at one end of the table. This was nuclear medicine's wonder of x-rays, but it looked much like a large commercial clothes dryer. The room was very cold and I shivered. Covering my torso and legs with a warm blanket, the technician said "I know it is cold here, Diane. However, we must have it this temperature for the equipment. Do you remember that?"

"Only vaguely," I sighed.

Slowly, the technician began moving my sliding examination table into the large cylinder. When my head was under the rim, the cylinder began spinning slowly, gradually picking up speed. I was instructed to hold perfectly still and breathe normally.

I felt very relaxed. As the machine completed its whirling and spinning, I experienced no sensation whatever. The technician advised me that the results of both tests would be available by mid-afternoon.

Although there had been nothing physically straining or uncomfortable about the two procedures, I was very tired from the emotional tension. When I reached home, I sank into my bed fully clothed, and quickly fell into a deep sleep.

I awakened with a start and looked at my clock. It was almost office closing time, and I had not called the neurologist for my test results. Quickly I retrieved his telephone number from my wallet, and dialed. His receptionist, a foreign woman with halting English, answered, and stated that the doctor wanted to discuss the results with me in his office, the next morning.

Well, thank goodness! It was encouraging that the doctor wanted to speak to me personally. Most people would probably see something negative in that, I figured. But not if you seriously had concerns about your sanity! I was not "losing my mind," as I had feared; there might be a little problem, but nothing too serious to talk about, I reasoned. Whatever was wrong, I certainly felt too physically fit for it to be anything dire.

The next morning I arrived at my neurologist's office in good spirits, with only a modicum of apprehension. He sat behind his cluttered desk and went over the results with me.

"Your EEG was basically the same as before, Diane, no new damage," he offered.

Before he could continue, I interrupted.

"What do you mean, 'no new damage?' I have no previous permanent damage."

"From the minor stroke you sustained, Diane," he stated slowly.

"You told me I had no permanent damage! I have noticed no permanent damage! I have had no symptoms of anything amiss until, well, until. . ." my voice trailed off.

"I am certain I explained to you before," my neurologist continued, smoothly. "You had some mildly abnormal reading from the right temporal lobe. It is nothing earthshaking, Diane, but it is what we refer to as an abnormal reading."

I felt a cold sensation in the pit of my stomach. I was absolutely certain that he had not advised me of any abnormality whatsoever. However, listen to the man, hear him out, I thought. This is not the time to rile your physician.

"Now, for your MRI examination, Diane. You know, this procedure is still relatively new, and there may be just a difference in the reading of your first MRI and the one conducted yesterday," he stated with an encouraging smile. "However, I went over to read it, looked at the film myself, and while it shows no sign of any lesion or tumor, no great anomaly, it does delineate some unidentified disparity in the white matter. I recommend that we do nothing as it probably means nothing, and that we continue on as we have. Just keep your nose clean."

I stared at him in frustration, attempting to absorb his words, wondering at his cavalier manner.

"Doctor, what are you saying? Nothing is wrong? Or there is something wrong?"

"I am simply stating that there is no great change from your previous tests, and therefore I see no reason to expect the worse. This has bothered you greatly, hasn't it, Diane?"

"Yes, it has bothered me greatly!" I exclaimed. "I lost four hours that wretched day! I drove who knows where, totally lost, in my own stamping ground, in what should have been a twenty-minute trip, maximum! I have been losing my balance, and not through dizziness, but rather as though someone was moving the ground beneath me. I cannot remember what I cooked for dinner last night. I make notes for anything and everything. Yes! Yes! I am bothered!" I paused.

"You know, Diane, perhaps you should see a psychologist, have some counseling, for your nerves," he said soothingly. "Are you taking the tranquilizer as directed?"

The clammy feeling in the pit of my stomach now spread throughout my body. He felt me to be a basket case, after all! I declined his offer of referral to a psychologist, arose, shook his hand and left the office.

At home, I tried to put the pieces together, but nothing fit. If my tests were not normal, then why wasn't I given a better explanation of what was happening? And why recommend a psychologist, if my physical tests were abnormal? Was it my nerves? Perhaps I was, without being aware of it, worrying entirely too much about my health. Resolutely, I decided to follow his instructions, take one day at a time, and "keep my nose clean."

Two months went by without incident. Then one day at work I had another frightening experience. I had worked diligently and under pressure to get a trial

17

brief transcribed before a deadline and was on my way
to deliver it to the attorney. As I entered the main corridor, the floor suddenly heaved and swayed, pitching
me against the polished marble wall. The ground
swirled and I clung to the wall until finally the plush
carpet was still and quiet.

I gingerly stepped away from the marble wall and
walked shakily to the attorney's office. Seeing the
transcript, he raised his hands above his head in a vic-
tory cheer, and smiled his appreciation. I stated that I
would be standing by for any changes or questions he
may have and returned to my secretarial office.

As I sat down behind my polished, glass covered
desk, a brightly dressed woman approached.

"Yes?" I greeted her. "How may I help you?"

"Diane!" the woman paused in obvious surprise.
"Whatever do you mean?"

I felt a throbbing in my chest as I realized the woman
thought we knew each other, and on a first-name basis.
But who was she?

Staring at me intently, the woman placed a sealed payroll envelope in front of me.

"Payroll came while you were delivering the brief transcript," the woman said slowly. "I took your paycheck
for you."

Obviously, this woman worked with me. I massaged
my temples, declaring a splitting headache, and
thanked the woman for keeping my paycheck. She
inquired if I had aspirin, and I nodded my head affir-

matively. With a puzzled expression, she left my office.

I needed to freshen up and arose and wandered silently through the work-space searching for the restroom. My office was open-plan, the law firm believing that only attorneys required privacy. There were no doors, just openings in the walls that led into corridors. I came to a corridor and walked down slowly, peering at the doors. No restroom, a dead end. I retraced my footsteps, and entered another hallway. This time, I struck pay dirt; straight ahead was the ladies' restroom. Inside I splashed cold water on my face, then dried myself carefully, so as not to smudge make-up. Examining myself in the large mirror, I looked fine. Nothing out of the ordinary.

As I entered the corridor, a well-dressed young man was turning the corner.

"Hey, Diane! Good to see you! How have you been?" he greeted me with a smile.

Oh God, not another one! I felt I was on a trip to never-never land. This time, I attempted to bluff my way through small talk with the young stranger. As we walked along together, he asked me how long I had worked for this firm. I hesitated, then replied I had been with them for about three years. The lad nodded approvingly, and said he was there to interview for a job as messenger or courier. Could I help him?

I threw in the towel, and smiled resignedly at him.

"Please forgive me. I know that I know you, but it is just one of those days! I simply can't bring your name to mind. I will be happy to put in a word for you, if you could write down your name and other relevant details."

"I don't get it," he muttered.

"Your name?" I did not waver.

"Diane, I'm your cousin, Rich," he said slowly.

Tears began to surface in my eyes, and I embraced my cousin, whispering, "I was just trying to keep anyone from overhearing that one of my relatives is applying. Of course I'll put in a good recommendation with the personnel department. Absolutely!"

It struck me that while I may forget relatives, co-workers, or the way to the restroom, I certainly could think fast enough when cornered, and come forth with a believable bluff.

After bidding my cousin farewell, I returned to my office and buzzed the personnel clerk on the intercom. Keeping my voice bright, I stated that I could vouch for the young man who had just applied for the "gopher" (go-for-anything) position. The clerk said she would send the necessary form to me via the inter-office memo route. That cheered me and I turned back to my word processor, happy to have salvaged something from the day's disaster. I reached forward to the keyboard, and as I did so, my world suddenly blurred. Losing consciousness, I fell forward, then slid off my chair to the floor.

When I came to, I could not see anything, nor could I move. However, I could hear voices which sounded as though they were coming through an echo chamber. Someone was stating they were getting no pulse.

Another voice was calling for anyone who knew cardiopulmonary resuscitation (CPR).

Then I was jarred into consciousness by a sharp pain as something hard was placed forcefully against my bosom. The echo chamber was gone, and I could hear clearly. I could also feel movement about me, something binding on my arm, tightly. I opened my eyes, and it appeared two blue uniformed auto mechanics were over me. I blinked, to clear my vision, and one of the 'auto mechanics' spoke.

"Hello, sleeping beauty! Diane, we are paramedics, and we are here to help you. Can you tell us what happened?"

I groaned and shook my head.

The paramedics went about their tasks, and I realized I had already been placed on a stretcher. They assured me that my vitals were now fine, but that they must transport me to the nearest hospital for observation.

I drifted in and out of consciousness as they carried my stretcher into the elevator, and loaded me into the ambulance outside the building.

When I next regained consciousness, I was in the emergency room, and a doctor was talking to Jack. Someone must have telephoned Jack! Now I was in for it!

The man in white asked if I knew what had happened to cause my "syncope." I didn't even know what "syncope" was. He explained I had suddenly lost consciousness at work, and for a short interval had registered such low pulse and respiration that CPR was administered and paramedics summoned.

I groggily tried to tell him of the heaving floor and of of how I couldn't recognize a relative and co-worker. My speech was slurred, even to my own ears.

"Do you take any drugs? What have you taken today?" the suspicious doctor queried.

"No!" I cried. "I take one tranquilizer in the morning, one at night, nothing else!" Then, remembering, I added, "And I forgot to take the one this morning."

He asked Jack if I might have ingested drugs. Jack's jaw muscles tightened as he refused to admit any such addiction on the part of his wife.

They left the room and shortly afterwards, Jack returned with the news that I must leave the hospital. It seemed that this facility was not approved by his company's insurance carrier, so I had to go. The doctor suggested I contact my neurologist, or perhaps go directly to an emergency facility approved by my insurance carrier. I asked to be taken home. I had had enough for one day. ↩

3

CHANGE OF DIRECTION

*N*ext morning, I telephoned my office to report that I was fine, but would require a few days off. Then, with a resigned sigh, I telephoned my neurologist's office and requested that his receptionist give me an emergency appointment for that same day. The receptionist confused me with another patient, and then inadvertently connected me with the doctor, who was awaiting another call. Briefly, I explained my episode of "syncope" (whatever that meant) at work, and requested an immediate appointment. He agreed.

I did not have to wait long before the neurologist escorted me once again into his office. After hearing my description of the previous day's events, he asked if I would now consider a psychologist.

I was perplexed.

"Look, doctor! I lost consciousness! Paramedics were called! I want to know what is happening to me. I did not recognize a co-worker, then a relative. I had another of the episodes of the floor heaving to and fro underneath me. Something is causing that!"

He frowned at me. "Don't you see how worked up you are about this, Diane? I really wish you would go see a friend of mine, great chap, really. He can no doubt make you feel much better."

I crumbled as tears surfaced in my eyes. I sat back in my chair and nodded my agreement to seek counseling from the "great chap."

After receiving a copy of my medical chart, the psychologist agreed to test me immediately. He first conducted a battery of multiple-choice questions which I had to answer on a multi-paged computer test form. Half-way through, I became confused with the double meanings of some of the questions, repetitions, and unclear jargon.

I labored to complete the test, but became so lost and overcome that I began crying. Embarrassed, I realized that this certainly would not look well on my sanity's behalf! I cowered inside the little stall in which I sat completing the test answers, considering ripping the papers into shreds.

Deciding against such a juvenile measure, I doggedly wiped the tears away and finished the test, no longer trying to answer with great accuracy. Just get something entered. Just get this thing over with!

Afterwards, the psychologist gave me a verbal test, then a set of motor coordination puzzle blocks to complete. The procedure took a total of three hours. Another testing appointment was scheduled for the next morning. I was exhausted.

The second day's testing began with additional motor coordination and word association. Then he handed me a piece of paper, and showed me a simple design, directing me to copy it onto my piece of paper. There were eight of these simple basic designs: square, cross, circle, square with diagonal line, circle with wavy line crossing, and other rudimentary shapes. After I had drawn the shapes onto my piece of paper, he removed the sheet and asked me to draw all the shapes from memory.

I tried to get as many sketched as I could, but knew from my own experience that I could not remember them all. Recently I had to request that callers repeat their telephone numbers as I could not remember the seven digits and write them down without a repeat. However, the psychologist told me I was doing well, thus far.

Next, he handed me some odd-shaped pieces of cardboard, six in all. There was one large, irregularly round piece, and five elongated pieces of varying lengths. I was to form a shape with the puzzle.

The puzzle stumped me. The psychologist tried to give me cloying hints. It was a thing. It was a part of my body. Try as I might, arranging and rearranging the pieces, I could not make a recognizable form from it. It was hopeless. Finally the psychologist quickly moved the pieces together in the shape of a hand. I sat stunned, looking at the simple cardboard hand, now so obvious.

Four blocks with white background and red mark across each came next. I was to arrange the blocks so that they formed a design.   Only four blocks! Make something! Anything! Even if wrong, he will judge you creative! I tried, becomingly increasingly nervous. Then I tried to give myself a mental pep talk. Finally, he laid a photo of the design before me.

"This is it, Diane. Make the blocks form this design."

It was still beyond me. He deftly reached over and moved the blocks into the simple design.

I was failing a great many of his tests, even though I had no great difficulty with motor or hand-eye coordination in my everyday life. I was still gainfully employed as an excellent, highly proficient legal secretary. Well, perhaps not so excellent as before. Perhaps not so proficient, either, I admitted begrudgingly to myself. Perspiration was beginning to form on my palms and my mouth was uncomfortably dry.

I did well with the addition and subtraction tests and began to relax. Maybe I was not too bad. The final phase came at last. The psychologist read a short paragraph, then asked me to answer certain questions about the content. Then he read a story, and asked me to repeat the general story line. As I triumphantly finished, he questioned me about the details. I drew a mental blank. Was he tricking me? I remembered none of those details being in the story he read.

Afterwards, I felt I had been put through a wringer, and could have killed for a good drag from a cigarette. I was in my third day of attempting to quit smoking in an effort to achieve better health. Once inside my car, I leaned back against the headrest for a few minutes and took a deep breath. Then I sat upright, uttered a string of expletives, and retrieved an unopened pack of cigarettes from its secret hiding place in my automobile. I sat, indulging my craving for nicotine, and smoked one all the way to the filter, then started the ignition and drove out of the parking lot.

The psychologist telephoned the following day with his opinions following my testing. "Diane, I really had hoped to determine that your symptoms were psychosomatically induced. However, there is a clear pattern here, and your problem is not in my ball park, but the neurologist's. Therefore, I am dictating a letter to him today, with a copy of the test results, recommending he conduct extensive blood tests, a brain scan, and other neurological tests to determine your exact condition."

"Please explain what you mean by a 'pattern,'" I asked, reaching for a cigarette, my sixth today.

"We can determine by our testing procedure where you have sustained neurological damage. That is a pattern which you cannot imitate, cannot fake, and cannot camouflage, Diane. So I am forwarding the test results and my recommendation for additional testing and a blood workup. Sometimes these things are masking a chemical imbalance, which also causes a loss of capacity. I am requesting your neurologist take another run at this."

I thanked the psychologist, and told him I would consider his offer of counseling.

A week later, I had still not heard from my neurologist regarding the additional testing which I was told was necessary. I made an appointment and cornered him in his lair. I was astonished that he said nothing about future tests, but instead recommended psychological counseling.

In exasperation I responded, "The psychologist informed me personally that he was recommending additional tests be conducted by you. He stated my only emotional problem is in attempting to cope with losses, and the lack of certainty as to cause," I bit the words off mincingly, crisply.

The neurologist raised his eyebrows in puzzlement.

"Diane, I am not ready to take directions from an individual with only a degree in psychology," he stated. "I want you to take an anti-depressant, additional dosage of the tranquilizer, and undergo counseling."

I decided against voicing my thoughts and arose from my chair. I walked out to the receptionist's office and requested a copy of my records. I would wait. Yes, even if it took all day, I would await them. I would pay for the photocopying. I had the statutory right to my medical records.

"Thank God, I still remember some things," I smiled ruefully.

I looked over the records to determine that they also included a copy of the psychologist's test results. Satisfied, I drove home, bitter, but determined in my resolve to take my own reins in hand.

Arriving home, I pored over my medical records. I had to re-read most of them, as I had difficulty absorbing the contents and terminology.

Now what was I to do? I knew I required another neurologist, one who would conduct an extensive battery of neurological tests and a blood profile. I flipped through the yellow pages. Suddenly, my eyes focused on the listing for the Alzheimer's Association in the Orlando area. Surely they would know the name of a reputable neurologist.

The answering voice was kind, polite and helpful. While they could not "recommend" a physician, per se, they could tell me the name of a doctor who worked closely with the Association, and was the neurologist for many of their patients. The kind voice asked for the symptoms, and who was the patient? I hesitated, and then stated the patient was a (non-existent) sister, and described then my own symptoms to the pleasant voice.

"You know, it sounds as though your sister may have Alzheimer's," the voice stated carefully.

"Oh, no!" I said. After thanking the woman for her assistance, I called Dr. T., the neurologist, and requested an appointment.

The earliest appointment I could get was for the following month. I was disappointed by the wait, but somehow, making the change in neurology services gave me a more positive outlook. Something was going to be done. I had my own reins in hand at last.

I returned to work in an upbeat mood, but within a few short days, my positive attitude crumbled. I was making mistakes on the job, and as a perfectionist, was annoyed at myself. I forgot to enter two important dates on the attorney's calendar. I kept forgetting where certain equipment or offices were located. Others had begun to notice and asked about my confusion.

It got gradually worse. One day I could not remember on which floor of the tall office building my office was located. Another day, I could not find my car in the parking garage and walked seven floors, scanning approximately sixty cars on each floor, until I found mine.

As it became more obvious to everyone at work that I was "not quite with it," I made the painful decision to resign my position. To get around my handicap and still stay employed, I decided to contact an agency specializing in temporary legal assignments. I figured that no one would expect a temporary assistant to know know her way around a building or office, nor recognize the employees on sight. If I erred, it would seem natural, nothing amiss.

Of course going to the new location each morning and arriving home each evening would be a problem, but I had already figured a way of coping with navigation difficulties. One day, having been forced to stop at a gas station to get my bearings around town, I noticed a tourist requesting directions. The clerk practically took the man by the hand and led him where he was going. Aha! Orlando is unfailingly polite to tourists, I thought. And thus I began introducing myself as "a tourist" when asking directions. Orlandoans gave much better directions to tourists than to locals, because they expected locals to be familiar with the territory.

My first temporary assignment went without a hitch. The small practitioner only wanted someone to answer his phone and greet clients. He was delighted that I also knew how to set up his files and take dictation. His parking lot was right outside his office door. No chance for me to get lost, there.

I was grateful I had the foresight to begin my tenure as a"glorified temp," as I referred to my new career venture. The temporary assignments afforded me the opportunity to work and maintain my self-esteem, and I was able to take off whenever required for medical appointments.

My increasing lack of familiarity with routine legal procedures and forms was very demeaning. However, I was relieved that the law offices to which I travelled did not question this.

At one time, I had managed a law office.

At one time, I had been a legal assistant, conducting research, traveling to court, doing administrative work, delegating duties to others, and overseeing office procedures.

At one time, I had acted as hostess on behalf of the senior partner of my law firm at a dinner party honoring the governor.

At one time, I had an IQ of 137. ☜✎

4

SECONDARY TESTING

*T*he days gradually passed and finally my first appointment with Dr. T., my new neurologist, was at hand. I sat in his waiting room, examining the wall hangings and counting the tiles in the ceiling. At last my name was called and I went in to meet my new specialist.

He was personable and had already read over my neurological and psychological records. After examining me thoroughly, we had a lengthy conference. I felt like kissing his hand in appreciation as he told me he would embark on a neurological examination and series of tests. There would be another EEG, another MRI, a brain scan, a complete blood work-up and a chemical profile. He wanted to perform a lumbar puncture (spinal tap) immediately. Dr. T. preferred not to extend an opinion without lab verification, but he wanted to hear my impressions.

I was taken aback. Faltering, I told him that I did not

know what was wrong, other than it was physical, and there "was less of me every day than there was the day before." I felt the small stroke was probably the culprit; but I did not understand the sudden increase in memory loss and directional problems.

Trying to appear competent, I confided that I had relearned, with great difficulty, traffic signals and signs. Feeling confident as he raised no eyebrow, I added that I had also relearned the simple directions of left, right, up, down, clockwise, counter-clockwise, over, under, and so on. I had them back in my memory, but had to consciously recall them. Following directions was no longer an automatic function.

Dr. T. sat in silence for a moment, gazing at me. Then he cleared his throat and complimented me on my tenacity and self-help methods. He said it reflected it a great deal about my own self image. I sighed in relief.

Then as I was leaving his office, I turned in the wrong direction and instead of arriving at the receptionist's station, walked into a closet.

After test results were in, the neurologist scheduled me for a conference with him. He announced that there were no problems with my chemical profile, lumbar puncture, and blood test. The EEG and MRI results were another story.

Dr.T. explained carefully that these tests indicated I had sustained damage in multiple quadrants of my cerebral vascular system. Quietly, he stated that while there was no way to undo the damage, nor regain the lost material, I should not relinquish my efforts to relearn. He stated positively that my brain scan results might be more encouraging, but at present it appeared I had sustained permanent damage to several small areas of the brain due to "multi-infarct," or multiple breakdowns within the brain's blood vessels. He also stated, to my dismay, that the condition was progressive.

I sat silently, not wanting to believe my ears. "Are you saying I will only get worse, never better? What can I do to stop it, slow it down, something?" I asked, lifting my face up to the ceiling and avoiding looking into his eyes.

"Avoiding stress would be helpful, but there is no cure. Ceasing smoking, well, it might slow deterioration by one to four percent, but again, there is no cure. For now, just live as happily and actively as you can. Keep your mind active. Attempt to relearn lost material. It is essential that you afford yourself mental stimulation as well as regular retreats of relaxation. Take trips. Visit friends. Enjoy life."

He had another topic to discuss.

"Diane, up until now you have displayed an excellent sense of humor. Don't lose it, at this point. Cling to it. That will help you keep a positive attitude about yourself and life in general. Positive attitudes help many people survive traumas."

I nodded my head in dumb acceptance.

"Another thing," the physician continued. "Is there any history in your family of others suffering from anything similar?"

"What?" I looked up in confusion.

"We have found a strong hereditary factor in these cases. I am not stating definitely that you have multi-infarct dementia. It could also be Alzheimer's Disease. It could be both. I don't want to scare you to death. I imagine you are already quite frightened. I know I would be."

I shook my head to his query as to hereditary factors. Then I gazed into his eyes piercingly.

"What did you say? Alzheimer's Disease? No!" I cried out.

"For now, just consider it a possibility. Do you want to know if it is, Diane?"

"*I want to know everything!*" I emphasized with my hands. "All! Whatever! Multi-infarct, Alzheimer's, each, both, whatever!"

I walked out of the neurologist's office numb. I had thought that this visit would dispel all my fears and help me regain my old self. Instead, he had just told me to hang on, hang tight, because the ride ahead could be rough. I drove home in an absent-minded daze, and got lost twice before negotiating my way into my own driveway. This time, however, I felt it was understandable.

I did not feel open to discussing the findings of the neurologist's tests with my husband. Jack had been small comfort about anything for several years. We had, in fact, fallen into the ignominious state of silence, except for such necessities as "I think the house is on fire."

35

I felt my house was indeed burning, but did not feel able to confide in my husband. Feelings of guilt and loneliness overwhelmed me and after a few days I decided to approach him about the findings related to my medical tests.

Jack frowned. "Just stop worrying about everything!" he insisted. "I don't worry, and I get by!"

"And that is why I worry!" I snapped defiantly. "And that is how you get by!"

Jack began waving his hands at me in agitation and annoyance. "And another thing! Stop smoking! I have been thinking about quitting, myself. Get off the cigarettes and you will improve a lot, Diane!"

"Don't yell at me about smoking tonight, Jack, please! I have had just about all I can handle, today."

"See?" he raised his arms toward the ceiling in desperation. "Perfect! You are going to worry about this nonsense until you drive yourself nuts!"

I retreated into the bedroom and stretched across the bed. My head was throbbing. I was probably going to fall into a migraine headache, on top of everything else. Resolutely, I called my friend, Elise, who had cheered me on many occasions when either my medical or marital tension was depressing me.

The sound of my friend's voice calmed me and I poured out all my fears and as much of the conversation with Dr. T. as I could remember verbatim. Then I paused, exhausted, for Elise to assimilate it all.

"Diane," she said sadly. "I didn't want to frighten you,

but this is just what I was afraid was happening. I recognized some of the symptoms."

But there is still the brain scan, I said, hoping against
hope. Elise offered to accompany me to the test
which was scheduled for the following week.

Although touched by my friend's offer, I declined. My
own husband had never accompanied me to a neurologist's office. He had never offered. When I needed
accompaniment, I would insist he perform some of
the husbandly role expected by society.

A week later, I arrived for the brain scan in better spirits. The assistant exchanged my clothing for a hospital
gown, and instructed me to lie down on the vinyl table
beneath a large box containing part of the sophisticat-
ed x-ray equipment. The cylinder at the head of the
table looked very much like the MRI "clothes dryer."

The technician affixed a blood pressure gauge to one
of my fingers, and inserted a needle into my arm to
begin an intravenous flow. She explained in a soft
voice the procedure: a radioactive dye would be injected through the intravenous tube, and then watched
via a console. As the dye flowed throughout my cerebral system, it would be photographed by the whirling
cylinder.

Soon the whirling cylinder was in action, and I closed
my eyes and tried to relax. There was no pain, no dis-
comfort. Only the disquieting reason for my being
there in the first place.

After the test, I dressed and left the outpatient clinic.
As I stepped into the bright sunshine of a typical
Florida day, on impulse I put the top down on my con-

vertible and drove home with the breeze blowing through my hair. It was a day perfect for white convertibles and ladies who drove them; ladies without a care in the world.

Upon arriving home, I had second thoughts about preparing dinner. I placed the thawing meat back into the refrigerator and telephoned Jack at his work station to tell him that he was taking me out to dinner that night.

"What's the occasion?" he asked. "And who is paying?"

"The occasion is starting to live instead of survive," I announced with verve. "And you can pay, Sugar Daddy!"

I hung up the phone with his laughter still ringing in my ears. Perhaps I needed to take this marriage by the reins, as well. While I could still hold them.

The following day, Dr. T's secretary telephoned with the results of the brain scan. Slowly, she stated that the results confirmed the diagnosis of dementia. If I had any questions, they would be glad to set an appointment.

No, I had no questions. I was too stunned. I hung up the phone and drove into town to begin a new temporary assignment.

Embarking on new assignments in unfamiliar offices was now causing me great difficulty. New surroundings, new people, new parking arrangements, new clients, all began to engulf me with paralyzing fears. This drive was harrowing and I had to stop three or four times for directions.

My new office was in a refurbished old building. One minute I was coping fine with my work. The next, I had lost complete recall of whom I was speaking to on the telephone, and why. An awkward silence elapsed, and the client began asking if I was still on the line. Confused, I asked him to hold for one minute, and pushed the designated "hold" button. Frantic, I tried to recollect the client's name and what we were discussing. I could not. I had not the slightest glimmer. Looking about my desk top for a sign of what the conversation might be about, I found no hint.

The attorney began buzzing for me, and another line was ringing. A short, chubby blonde woman wearing heavy make-up entered my office and collapsed heavily into a chair. I had no idea who she was. What did she want? The attorney now shouted impatiently for me.

Shakily, I arose from my desk and went to the attorney's office. He demanded to know what was happening? Why were all the lines ringing?

I swayed as I held onto the back of an overstuffed chair near his desk. "I am very ill, and must leave, immediately," I whispered. "Right now. I am very sorry. I will have the agency send you someone else."

Before his startled gaze, I picked up my purse and fled his office. Seeking safety in the familiar confines of my car, I sat for a few minutes before starting the engine. Then with a pang, I realized I could not negotiate my way out of the parking lot. Everything looked the same. It was like being in a maze. I had become disoriented many times in parking garages, and on numerous occasions in stores I found myself turning around in a tight circle, as all aisles appeared to be identical. This was the first time it had occurred in a parking lot; a small parking lot.

I turned off the engine and leaned back against the head rest, closing my eyes and taking a deep breath. After a while, I restarted the motor, and slowly circled the parking lot repeatedly, until I found an opening. Then I drove over a curb to get to the street.

Arriving home without incident, I prepared a hot bubble bath. The drapes were still drawn and the house was dark but I let it be. I undressed, letting my garments stay on the floor where they landed. I eased myself into the steaming, fragrant bubbles, and soaked my cares away. Leaning back against the smooth tub, I slid down until my chin was at the bubble level and some bubbles even tickling my nose. Closing my eyes, I remained in my refuge for over an hour.

The Alzheimer's Association had been forwarding literature to me which I immediately cast into the trash without reading, as though they were pornographic, repugnant. However, as though directed by an all-knowing entity, another pamphlet had come in today's mail, and this time I did not discard it unread.

I read through the articles on the disease as I lay stretched across my bed. I had not bothered to dress after my bath, and my satin comforter felt smooth, cool and heavenly to my bare skin. Suddenly, my attention focused on a small article describing a new testing procedure for diagnosing Alzheimer's Disease. My pulse quickened as I read of this test, designated only as SPECT, another marvel of the nuclear age of medicine. Through this new procedure, isotopes, which demonstrate clearly which type of dementia is present, if any, could be isolated.

Normally, Alzheimer's disease could only be diagnosed for certainty by autopsy after death. Now this new testing procedure could isolate and delineate the rare isotopes in even early cases of dementia.

I telephoned the neurologist's office. I did have some questions, now. The office scheduled me for an appointment the next day. I noticed that now I was a bona fide patient, I did not have to wait long for an appointment with Dr. T.

Immediately upon his entrance into my examining room, I began reading aloud from my notes regarding the SPECT test. Dr. T. stated the test was rather new on the market, and, as such, may not be entirely reliable. I looked at him beseechingly.

"Please. I have to know. Please."

Then I told him of my aborted work assignment at the law office, of burned pot holders and dish cloths, twelve in all. I showed him the burns on my wrists and arms sustained because I forgot to protect myself when inserting or removing food from the oven. I told him of becoming lost in the neighborhood grocery where I had shopped for over twenty years. I showed him my scribbled notes and sketched maps of how to travel to the bank, the post office, the grocery, and work.

Tears began to flow as I told him of how distressed I was at the way I had "gone up" when I became confused and disoriented at work. Of my difficulty exiting the small parking lot.

"You know, Diane, I really think it is time you ceased trying to work," he said gently, as I paused for breath. "I am recommending you retire."

I stopped short, shocked. "I am too young to retire," I stated flatly.

"I was thinking along the lines of a disability. I think you should apply. You have tried to carry on a remarkably long while. It is time you rested, took care of yourself."

"I would never qualify for a disability," I protested. "I am not that... that disabled," I finished lamely.

"I am directing that you cease work immediately. My God, you have stretched this out remarkably. It is time to stop."

"No," I stated emphatically. "I still have 'miles to go before I sleep,' Dr. T. See? I remember that! I even know who wrote it! Robert Frost! See?"

The neurologist made a pact with me. He would order the requested SPECT test if I would consider ceasing work. He then added one comment to haunt me.

"Diane, if you don't want to think of fairness to yourself, think of fairness to others. Persons for whom you go to perform duties you can no longer perform."

"Okay," I nodded. "I will think about it. But if not a legal secretary, surely there are other jobs I could do. Clerk in a little card store, maybe? I enjoy all kinds of greeting cards. Perhaps?"

His eyes were kindly as he smiled slowly and said I deserved an "A" for effort, but surely I knew, deep down, that I could not log sales, I could not make change, I could not handle money easily. However, he would schedule my SPECT test, and when the test results were in, he would speak with me again about termination of my employment, and filing for disability benefits.

When I arrived for the SPECT test, I had difficulty locating the correct lab. Twice I asked directions and attempted to follow them. Finally, a woman wearing the pink hospital volunteer uniform assisted me and led me directly to the laboratory.

I had to wait thirty minutes before the test could begin. Due to my difficulty with directions, I usually left for a destination with at least an hour to spare, to allow myself sufficient time to perhaps be lost and then get my bearings.
During my wait, my bladder became painfully full. I did not want to go to the restroom, as I could probably not find my way back. Finally, I could not bear the full bladder any longer, and approached the lab receptionist.

"I have difficulty with directions. Could you please give me directions to the nearest restroom?"

The receptionist obliged with simple, two-step instructions. I became lost, asked another person for directions, and finally entered the restroom with a sigh of relief. After exiting the restroom, I attempted to retrace my steps back to the lab, but became hopelessly lost in a maze of corridors. Then I feared I was not even on the same floor, although I did not remember leaving the lab floor.

An older, white-haired lady wearing the hospital uniform was approaching. Biting back tears, I stopped the woman. "Please help me," I admitted in a whisper. "I am a dementia patient and cannot find the lab for. . ." I showed the woman my note specifying the name of the test and the room number.

"Oh, my goodness! Are you alone? Is no one with you?" the woman exclaimed, shocked. "Didn't someone bring you here, today?"

I fought the desire to shout, "Yes, yes, I came here all by myself, just like a big girl!" Instead, I pressed my note into the woman's palm. She hastily took me by the arm and escorted me to the lab office, where she entered and spoke briefly to the personnel.

This test was a lengthy procedure, and required a little more cooperation from me than the previous tests. I was lying on the vinyl table, my chin strapped against my chest to prevent my head moving during the procedure. An attendant stood by as the large overhead x-ray camera circled about my head. Intravenous dye was again injected into my arm as preparation for the test.

A second attendant operated a computer with a console screen which showed colored plates of different parts of my cerebral area. The attendant was keying in instructions both to the camera and to the computer as the technique was administered.

Suddenly, the restraining strap broke. The test could not be halted, so they restrained my head again, chin against my chest, while the machine continued to turn and click. The procedure took approximately one hour, and my neck was hurting due to the prolonged uncomfortable position. The test was finally completed, and I was a free woman, again.

•   •   •

I waited impatiently for the results of the SPECT test. Dr. T. wanted to thoroughly review the plates and film as well as the report, before discussing the results with me. Finally the test results arrived. I tore the envelope open in haste, and read his report.

The "rare" isotopes had been found in my brain. The radiologist determined this to be proof of Alzheimer's Disease and multi-infarct dementia. Dr. T. cautioned, however, that due to the newness of the testing procedure, he was reluctant to pronounce me with such a severe diagnosis at this point. ❧

5

FRIENDS FOR ALL SEASONS

*I*t was a day of finality, my senses numbed, when I received the following letter from my treating neurologist. He had been reluctant to advise me of my completed diagnosis until I was undergoing counseling to enable me to cope with my situation.

Dear Diane:

As we have previously discussed extensively, it is my impression that you are suffering from dementia. The probability is that this is due to Alzheimer's disease. This is based on the findings of the studies we have done, clinical examination and probability statistics.

If I can be of any help in getting you into a research program, I would be glad to do so.

Respectfully submitted,

R.S.T., M.D.
Neurology Associates

I was devastated. At such a time, it is the blessed person who has a trusted friend or loved one to whom he or she can turn and receive comfort, empathy and solace, paired and coupled with a positive viewpoint. I no longer had that trusted friend and confidante.

My dear friend, Elise, had died one month previously. She had endured a blessedly short battle with melanoma, a vicious type of cancer. I had been able to return Elise some of the many comforts she bestowed on me, as I assisted her family in caring for her.

I knew that Elise was now relieved of any suffering, and therefore "better off," but selfishly wished I could have one more cozy exchange of confidences over a steaming cup of herbal tea. Wistfully, I went to the kitchen cabinet to prepare my own favorite raspberry tea. I would have this cup in memory of Elise. As I reached for the raspberry brew, I paused, and smiling, instead retrieved Elise's favorite choice, a blend of orange and spices.

Thinking of my dear departed friend, I prepared the cup of tea and carried it and the letter from Dr. T. into my bedroom. Not ready to discuss this development with anyone, if not Elise, I carefully hid the letter from my husband. I never knew how Jack would react to bad news. Usually he was as much of a morale boost as a rubber crutch to a broken leg.

I took my cup of tea into the bathroom and prepared a steaming bubble bath. Relaxing in the fragrant water and sipping my tea, I pondered how much my life had changed in the past few years, since my neurological troubles began. I had rounded the corner of a half century and now was approaching my fifty-third birthday. Morbidly, I wondered what changes would

occur within the next few years. There was so much to
absorb and digest, and my ability to do this was lessen-
ing each day.

I had become increasingly more selective in my
acquaintances. My husband and I had been having
sufficient marital difficulties that we no longer had
"couples friends," as we had enjoyed years before. I
had become particularly selective in making new
friends, due to fear of my memory and directional
problems being discovered.

I was playing a game of "I've Got A Secret" with everyone, even with myself. Still outgoing, quick to strike
up conversations with strangers, and thriving on a
good laugh, I was careful not to let my guard slip. I
must never let any acquaintance become too close, too
familiar. The expression "a little knowledge can be a
dangerous thing," took on new meaning to me. I did
not want outsiders to know me too well. By keeping a
safe distance, they would not discover my growing
weaknesses.

I finished my cup of tea, and exited the tub. Drying
myself, I moved, as was my habit, directly into the
bedroom, to lie stretched out luxuriously on my pale
blue satin comforter and rest for a while in the cool
room. My gaze rested on the stack of unopened mail
lying beside me on the bed. I was now reading the
pamphlets sent periodically by the Alzheimer's Association, to determine if any additional breakthroughs
were published that might assist me.

Idly, I flipped through the stack, dividing generic or
"junk" mail from the first class envelopes. Then I saw the
envelope from someone named Davidson, postmarked
in the small town in Ohio where I had grown up.

I opened the letter and was delighted to read that it was from my own childhood best friend, Marie Thomerson, now Marie Davidson.

"Dear Diane," the letter read. "I found your address in some old papers I inherited from our much beloved former Scout leader. In today's world of moving places and faces, I know I have a ninety percent chance of this letter being returned, 'Addressee Unknown,' but if you are the former Diane Friel, and you do receive this note, please write me. I am the former Marie Thomerson, and would love to hear from you."

I smiled, and immediately penned an reply.

"Dear Marie, Congratulations! You made the top ten percent at last! I am still here, and it was a delightful surprise in an otherwise wretched day to hear from you."

I briefly continued to tell her about my marriage, the names and ages of my children and two grandchildren, and my career history. I deliberately avoided any mention of medical history.

But her letter cheered me up and I dressed in haste and immediately drove to the post office to post my reply to Marie.

Marie and I had shared many wonderful childhood memories. Together we picked daffodils in the spring, made mud pies and played with holly hock dolls in the summer. In the autumn we were architects and builders of elaborate leaf houses, laying out great floor plans, and rolling with mirth in the tangy fragrance of the piles of multi-colored leaves. During Ohio winters, we made snow men, snow angels and snow ice cream.

Our favorite pastime, however, was the Saturday matinee features at the small town's movie theater. We thoroughly enjoyed them all, but the outstanding favorites were the musicals. After each feature we would act out the various parts, and sing and dance our hearts out.

I recalled with a wave of laughter the day Marie and I had viewed "Singing in the Rain," a lively musical starring Gene Kelly, Donald O'Connor, and Debbie Reynolds. When we exited the theater, it was into a downpour. Undaunted, we two had danced and pranced along the puddled walks and curbs, singing boisterously every song which had been performed in the feature until it was time to part ways to walk to our individual homes.

Gene Kelly had performed excellently choreographed dance routines in the movie, which included dancing along a puddled street through gutters, splashing and kicking in his wild song and dance, and swinging around lamp posts. The one thing my street did not lack was an abundance of both lamp posts and deep puddles during a heavy rain. By the time I arrived home, my Mary Jane blue suede shoes were ruined, and my clothing and hair were dripping their own puddles beneath my dancing feet. My mother was outraged.

My mother had tried hard to turn me into a silk purse, but I had been perfectly content to remain a sow's ear. Mother had taught me all the etiquette and manners required of a young lady, coached me in walking up and down a staircase while balancing a book on my head for posture and grace, and had also encouraged me to take dance, classical piano and voice lessons. My laughter faded as I remembered my mother even taking in ironing to pay for my vocal coaching. And for what? The only benefits gleaned from the years of lessons were that I had an intense appreciation of music and dance.

Another smile was tugging at my lips as I remembered my mother's shock when she learned that as an adult, I had undertaken belly dancing and was performing in a local restaurant which featured such entertainment. It was excellent exercise, however. I had been blessed with a genetic foundation that kept me slim, but the belly dancing kept me trim and youthful in muscular tone and spirit.

Memories made me feel good. Still on my nostalgic trip, I went into the spare bedroom and began looking through the photographic memorabilia of my dancing days. I sighed as I looked at the days gone by. What was, was!

I glanced through the photographs, and stopped at one of my mother. It had been several years since cancer had taken her from the family. It was bitterly unfortunate that she had died while still relatively young.

I moved over to my mother's cedar chest which now stretched the width of the foot of the double bed. I gently opened the chest and began looking through her belongings. Stored in the cedar scented protection were many memories which came flooding back. My hands rested on a small box I had packed inside the chest after my mother's death. It contained papers which I had not wanted to discard and had neatly packed away with my mother's other belong-

ings. Opening the box, I removed childhood draw-
ings my brother and I had made for mother, and little
sachet containers I had hand sewn for her.

Then I noticed the maps. After mother's death I had
found mysterious hand drawn maps and bits of directions scribbled on note papers all over her home.
They were in her purses, in bureau drawers, in the
desks, seemingly everywhere. Too distraught at the
time to figure out their purpose, I had simply packed
them all away with the other articles in the box.

Now I smoothed out each map and scrawled note, and
placed them side by side. They covered the bedroom
floor. There were maps to every place my mother
went about town, even to my home and to my brother's home. As I deciphered each note and map, I
began recollecting my mother's other eccentric habits.
She would not drive out of her neighborhood. She
would not drive at night. She was teased by both
myself and my brother about "memory goofs" and
would become very irate with both of her children
over their loving teasing.

Then with a chill, I recalled one day when I
approached my mother to tell her something, and
she did not recognize me.

I arose from the mementos and walked into my own
bedroom, where I pulled out my notebook of daily
reminders. Thumbing back through the entries, finally coming to the entry where Dr. T. had inquired of
any hereditary link relating to my neurological difficulties. I had said no. Now I wondered. Could it be
that my mother had begun to display the same symptoms and no one, not even her two children, had
observed or been shrewd enough to know there was a

problem?

I considered Dr. T.'s repeated instructions to have a family conference and advise my children of my situation. So far, I had not followed them. I could not bring myself to confide in my children. I could not even accept it myself. Intellectually, I knew my condition was not cause for shame, yet emotionally I felt ashamed. I was losing my intelligence, losing my memory, and my directional system was really shot to Hades.

Embarrassment kept me from confiding in my family and friends. I had no idea of how they would respond. If they were too condescending and made me feel totally worthless, I would chafe; on the other hand, if they displayed a "so what" attitude, I would be devastated. It would break my heart.

I wished I could unload this burden, reveal my thoughts to someone, state my innermost fears and anxieties, and receive kind support and understanding.

I did not know how my husband would take being forced to look at the situation clearly. He would need to know, soon. My income had been drastically cut when I began working part-time. What about the day when I could no longer get an assignment, even part-time?

What I wanted, no, needed, was someone to assure my that no matter what my future held, they would stand beside me, fight my battles with me, or if need be, for me. I wanted assurance from someone that I would not be abandoned to shrivel away. They would give me encouragement, love, moral support, and if necessary, take care of me.

I shivered in spite of myself.

Gently, tenderly, I repacked my mother's secret notes and maps back into the box, and carefully replaced it inside the cedar chest. ☜

6

RENEWAL

*M*arie, my childhood friend, and I began a flurry of correspondence, exchanged photographs, video tapes, audio cassettes, and long distance telephone calls too numerous for either budget.

We were ecstatic to discover that we still had the same strong rapport as when young. Each brought the other friend up to date on our lives, past and present, and of our hopes for the future. We shared reminiscences and fantasies. As laughter and tears bonded the two of us together again, I still could not divulge to Marie my marital discord or the presence of my medical situation.

I told Marie of my marriage to Jack McGowin, and gave her detailed accounts of each of my three children and two grandsons. Marie related her own marriage to David Davidson, and her rearing of not only her own four children but also over the years having played a role as foster parent to a total of nine other children. Marie also was a grandmother, to "three and one-half" children.

Marie and Dave were planning to move to Colorado in a couple of years, when he could effect an early retirement. They were going to drop out of civilization and Ohio, and into flannel shirts, boots and a mountain cabin to spend the remainder of their days. I averred I would stay the rest of my life in Florida, loving the sub-tropical breezes, great beaches, and year-round roses.

"Do you know how cold a Colorado mountain cabin will be? I pick bananas from my trees in the winter," I volunteered. "Roses all year, also."

Marie only laughed and said I would have to come out and visit and see what the mountains were really like, after she and Dave made the big exodus.

We planned to visit each other. I wanted to show Marie my favorite beach, the jetties at Ponce Inlet. Marie wanted me to see my own home town, and how it had changed.

I also wanted to see my old home town. The pilgrimage had long been on my mind. I longed to see old friends, and walk the streets I had known as a child. I wanted to touch again the Diane Friel who had once been, before she was no more.

As time passed, I wondered if I could divulge my neurological situation to Marie. The prospect appalled me, as I feared it would put a blight on our very upbeat relationship. However, it might be best that Marie be aware that any reunions should be affected earlier, not later. Later might be too late. I had no timeframe. The neurologist could not, or would not, give a time prognosis. That was entirely in the hands of God. I might have twenty more years to have get togethers with friends; on the other hand, I might not have twenty months.

Gradually, as my working days became fewer, I intimated to Marie that I had a few problems and required "more rest and time off than the average bear." Best to give it to her in doses, I thought. I did not want to risk losing my renewed friendship with the soul mate of my youth.

As a surprise, Marie forwarded to me a booklet distributed to the other former classmates from our home town. Various graduates had authored essays or anecdotes contained in the booklet. Marie had penned a note, "Be sure to read Kurt Fuller's article!" Obediently, I eased into my favorite easy chair and began reading the entries of all my former classmates.

When I reached the writings of Kurt Fuller, I smiled in fond reminiscence at the memories he recounted, many of which I also shared. Kurt, myself and another little boy, James Barber, had formed the Three Musketeers and had many great and not-so-great adventures together. The two boys had conspired to take advantage of my phobia of heights, and had literally launched me like a little curly-haired torpedo down the "big slide" at our elementary school.

After James and I had viewed a movie involving "blood brothers," I had persuaded him to perform the same bloodletting ritual with me, to become my blood brother.

On another occasion, Kurt, who was usually the mastermind in the boys' pranks upon me, had committed the most outrageous act of all. During a third grade class, Kurt had begun entertaining me with contortions of his face into hideous shapes. I sat entranced, giggling appreciatively as he became more and more extreme in his performance. Suddenly, Kurt leaped from his seat beside me and planted an amateurish eight-year-old boyish kiss on my startled mouth.

As I read Kurt's remembrances of victories on and off the athletic field, in and out of the scholastic arena, I suddenly froze in disbelief. He had written a humorous but pro-Kurt, anti-me accounting of that first kiss. It was his description of me as a child that sent me reeling.

"She wore round-lensed glasses, walked pigeon-toed and had jouncy sausage-shaped curls."

I fired a missal missile back at my third grade lover, giving my own rendition of that first kiss, and forwarded copies to the other former classmates who had received his published version.

To my surprise, a few days later Kurt telephoned me. We enjoyed many boisterous laughs over the "good ol' days." Kurt was now a professional writer, and had recently moved from Washington, D.C., where he had for many years held a position in the Capitol, to a new writing assignment in New York City. We, too established a routine of corresponding.

One evening Kurt telephoned to announce that he was closing his home in Washington D.C., and taking advantage of the empty house to hold an Honor Society reunion. Also, he had approximately nine hundred books remaining to be packed, the house

needed a "top-cleaning" sufficient to permit a paint
crew to be scheduled later that month. Would I
come? Would I help?

Leave it to Kurt! Always an angle! Nonetheless, I was
honored to be invited, and hesitated very slightly
before accepting. I knew the trip would be good for
me. And I wanted to see Kurt again. Gifted with high
intelligence, an incredible wit and twinkling eyes, Kurt
had always been my hero. I had been confident, no
doubt about it, that Kurt would be president one day.
This had caused much jesting and jeers from my fellow classmates, but I was convinced. Now I wanted to
see if I could "pass" in Kurt's eyes. I wanted to see if I
could meet the muster required within the intelligent
set of which I had once been a charter member. I
needed to see if I could pass the test.

I arranged for a through-flight so that I would not be
at risk during a plane transfer, and Kurt had volunteered to meet my plane. He would make reservations
for me at a hotel near his home. My days would be
spent socializing, packing books and other articles,
and removing dust. He had not cleaned the house
since his divorce twelve years prior. I packed casual
clothes and house cleaning apparel according to
Kurt's instructions, and flew to D.C. to see the
Musketeer in need.

My plane was delayed four hours due to bad weather.
Kurt, however, was true to his word and standing at
the gate as I disembarked. I was touched deeply as he
thrust a bouquet of roses toward me, stating, "Diane,
these are for you!" in much the manner of a shy little
boy thrusting a floral tribute forward. Then he
grabbed my arm and rushed me to the baggage pick-
up area. I cried out for him to wait a moment, I want-

ed to take a good look at him. It had, after all, been decades since we had seen one another.

I would have known him anywhere. Age had not spared him in countenance, but he had taken excellent care of himself. Kurt's mind and intellect were soon proved even more impressive than when a youth. He still had a ready sense of humor and love of a good time, but was so hyper he seemed just one jump ahead of a fit. He reminded me of the Mad Hatter in Alice in Wonderland. I was surprised to realize that I still held Kurt in the same high regard as so many years ago.

There was one new aspect to his personality, however. He now had a reserved dark side, a walled area with no trespassing into the inner Kurt. Well, don't we all? I laughed to myself. Although we shared many personal memories and private aspirations in our discussions over the next few days, I did not take Kurt into my private walled area, either, regarding my medical situation.

I was still nervous whether I could "get by" in strange surroundings with persons unaware of my "condition." Alone in the hotel at night, I became lost in the labyrinth of corridors, look-alike doors in the many-storied building. Often I had to seek assistance in locating my room. I slept with the light on each night.

On one occasion I stepped outside Kurt's Capitol Hill residence and decided to go for a short walk, simply to view the front of his home. I walked around the corner but upon my return, all house fronts appeared foreign to me. Which one was his? Just as I was fighting tears of frustration and was stiff with fear, Kurt found me. He had missed me in the house and had come

searching for me. I was never so glad to see anyone.
How kind and gallant of him to come looking for his
missing guest!

I admitted to Kurt that I had become lost on a little
walk, and he raised an eyebrow, stating if I were going
to pull stunts like that, he would put a leash on me.

"That will probably be next," I thought to myself and
apologized for causing him any concern; it had been
quite thoughtless of me to leave the building without
advising anyone. I never did again, for the duration of
my stay, without Kurt.

All in all, it was an enjoyable visit, and I was deeply
grateful to my host for his chivalry and kindness. I
had never felt as secure and safe as when in Kurt's
presence. I mused that I was probably still seeing him
as the Musketeer of valor I had envisioned him to be
when we were young.

There was one rough spot, during a discussion of various artists and authors. Kurt proudly showed me an oil
painting in his collection which was the work of the
wife of William Faulkner. When I did not realize that
Faulkner's wife was an artist, Kurt began to explain
who William Faulkner was. At his patronizing explanation, I snapped that "I knew ol' Bill well enough,"
but did not know his wife had been an artist. I could
tell from his surprised look that Kurt was perplexed by
my defensive reaction.

I was contrite. He probably thought me a dimwit. An
honor student gone to seed.

In a late night rap session which began to wax philo-
sophical, I referred to missing the "real Diane Friel,"

and when asked where I believed "the real Diane Friel" was, I replied simply, "She is dead." Kurt did not understand, and I did not elaborate. Instead, I beseeched him to never change, to which he replied sharply that people never change; no one he knew had ever changed. As a wave of overwhelming resentment, sorrow, fear and pent-up frustration enveloped me, I could say nothing more, and in lieu of words embraced Kurt tenderly. I knew he did not understand, but it really didn't matter. I understood.

The last day of my visit, Kurt was preoccupied with packing as I prepared to go to the airport. I kicked off my high heels and helped load additional boxes into the car before I wedged my suitcase and myself in with them. Kurt abruptly let me out of the car at the parking lot of the airport. I panicked, not even knowing which doorway to enter. I tried to handle my luggage and maneuver my way to my flight. I asked directions twice and finally a uniformed guard sensed something was amiss. As he walked me to the gate, I realized I was the last passenger boarding.

Once airborne, I began reflecting on my visit. All in all, I felt I had "passed." There were some "close calls" which had frightened me, but no one realized my fears except myself, and no misfortune befell me. I considered myself a success. I was learning to find joy in small victories, performing simple functions that were done by rote by most others.

Life could be worse. I still had a lot going for me. And there was still the possibility that my neurological deterioration could be slowed or stopped. And if not, I would have to learn to savor the friendships and loves I had been permitted to enjoy.

Turning these thoughts over, I looked out my window at the metropolis below. As I did so, the pilot announced that we were flying over Houston, Texas! My mind went numb and my throat tightened in fear. I had boarded the wrong aircraft!

Then, thankfully, the pilot apologized for his error and stated we were above Orlando, Florida. I had survived another close call. ᑌᗒᑕ

7

EARLY RETIREMENT

My next month was unbearably difficult at the workplace. Several times I became confused and disoriented and had to leave the office early. Life had become an improvisational theater, and I was left to ad lib my way through it. My doctor was still admonishing me not to work. I was still resisting. But it was becoming more difficult for me to function, or even find my way to work and back again.

At home, meals, pot holders, dishcloths and my arms were being burned. When attempting to prepare a simple recipe, sometimes luck was with me, more often not. I had lost weight I could ill afford to lose, and was beginning to suffer from insomnia. I sometimes lost my thread of thought in mid-sentence. Memories of childhood and long ago events were quite clear, yet I could not remember if I ate that day. On more than one occasion when my grandchildren were visiting, I forgot they were present and left them to their own devices. Moreover, on occasions when I had picked them up to come play at my house, the small children had to direct me home. Worst of all, my patience was nil. Much as I loved the children, I became anxious or nervous after just a short visit.

I contacted the Society for the Right to Die and obtained a Living Will. This would enable me to refuse life support systems or other "heroic" procedures in the event of impending death. I had to consider the possibility that some day, at some point in time, the Living Will might be needed by my family. However, I procrastinated in signing it. It was such an admission that I might become a burden to my family at some point in the future. I would fill it in at a later date. In the meantime, it would remain hidden away with the letter from Dr. T. advising me of the probability of my suffering from both Alzheimer's Disease and multi-infarct dementia.

To raise my spirits and self-esteem, I had plastic surgery to rejuvenate my eyelids. I was now desperately clinging to the belief that if I looked younger outside, my inside might be fooled.

After my eyelid surgery, I had to stay in bed and be cared for, as I could not see and was in pain. I was most grateful that Jack, who never previously displayed any concern or tenderness when I was undergoing surgery or ill, came through royally for me on this occasion. He saw to my needs kindly and with tender care. I was so appreciative of every small act of service that I was effusive in my praise of him.

Perhaps he would come through for me in the years ahead, should my capacities worsen. This was the first indication I had that I would be taken care of with kindness if I were to deteriorate. I needed that reassurance desperately.

I had still not followed Dr. T.'s repeated instructions to have a family conference and advise my kin of the situation. I was still afraid of how they would react; yet I still wished I could unload this burden.

Finally, at Dr. T's insistence, I gathered my family together to tell them about my illness. Everyone was there apart from my father, who was ailing, and my daughter Lynn, who resided in Tennessee.

My children were the most troublesome to tell. The two eldest, Bill, thirty-four, and Lynn, twenty-nine, were always the more masked in their emotions. I had frequently wondered if, indeed, my firstborn even had deep emotions for non-mechanical entities.

Then I would remember Bill as a child, always the quiet, tender one, always loyal and forever helpful. Yes, I thought, the emotions are there. Somewhere along the line, he chose to don a mask, perhaps due to so very much emotionalism and frenetic personalities surrounding him within our family.

My family's reactions were predictably quiet. But I was surprised by their stoicism and acceptance; an acceptance so very calm and cool that I wondered if it was actually non-acceptance. Shaun, my youngest, vehemently challenged the correctness of the medical evaluations, and told me: "Just don't worry about it, Mom; don't think about it." Bill said nothing. My daughter-in-law said I shouldn't have anything to worry about "for a long time."

My brother Charles expressed dutiful concern. His wife expressed greater concern for her husband, inasmuch as he had been having "considerable difficulty with memory lapses." I wanted him to have a conference and examination by my neurologist. He refused, stating he would look into that possibility when he "showed the same severe symptoms as you."

My husband stated I needed to "get my act together and just rise above all this."

When I arrived in Tennessee to tell Lynn, I was expecting more reaction. Instead, she accepted the news quite easily. I felt suspicious and asked my daughter if she had perhaps already suspected. Lynn smiled shyly and said well, no, but she had talked to Shaun.

"On the telephone. I just asked him, 'Shaun, how is Mom doing lately,' and he said, 'Same nut as ever, and you know how bad that is.'" Lynn's face broke into a teasing smile.

By now I knew my children were all getting quite a lot of mileage in jokes about me and my "little school friends," with jests flying hot and heavy among my offspring. But this was the first time I knew they had been keeping Lynn apprised of my medical status. They all knew I was slipping away.

Having always been the outspoken extroverted pivotal center of both my family and group of friends, I was now reluctantly in the non-contributing purgatory of the early diagnosed. I was discouraged by my family's individual stoic reactions. Perhaps I had not been as much of a contributing nucleus as I had egotistically thought!

The day finally came when I could not function on my job. My world was disintegrating and I had no platform on which to have a firm footing. Jack came home and found me in the darkened house, curled up in bed, fully dressed. I refused to tell him that I had finally reached my limit, stretched myself as far as I could.

He demanded that I explain my silent withdrawal. I feared his reaction. I felt worthless enough. Another vote in that direction from Jack, with his knack for cold, hurtful remarks, might well cave me in. I couldn't tell him.

At my next routine examination, the neurologist confirmed that my working days were over. It was time for my "early retirement." That night, I finally psyched up sufficient nerve to tell Jack that I could no no longer work.

"What is the doctor saying? That you are going to become a babbling idiot?"

His words cut through my heart and mind like a knife. My worse fear had been put into words.

Jack later apologized for the remark, and I accepted his apology. But the wound remained.

I told no one else that I had stopped working. I felt guilty that I could not function and was ashamed of my loss of capacities. My guilt was heightened as my father repeatedly telephoned and asked how I was enjoying my job, what days I had off, and other leading questions. I had never been a deceitful person. Now I was being deceitful to my father.

Then my daughter-in-law began dropping by "because your car was in the driveway." Now I worried that my married son and daughter suspected I was no longer working. Jack confirmed my fears.

"They are waiting for you to say something," he advised.

Lynn telephoned occasionally and often referred to my career. She was studying legal courses in college and frequently asked my opinion about certain details or regaled me with amusing stories. I could not tell her I'd quit working.

My son Shaun was moving out of our home and was preoccupied trying to find a reasonable yet fantastically plush apartment. He seemed oblivious to the fact that I was not working. His schedule frequently did not afford us so much time at home together and he was probably unaware that I was not leaving the house at all.

Now I felt I was deceiving all of my children.

Strangely enough, the two persons I did tell I was no longer working were Kurt Fuller and Marie Thomerson. I broke the news by letter, without revealing the cause; I referred to it as early retirement.

After all, that was the term my neurologist used with smooth psychology. I felt I had two close friends in Marie and Kurt. That they lived far away was a mixed blessing; I was greatly frustrated if their correspondence was late but the distance between us was a buffer against them realizing my difficulties.

I surely did appreciate Marie and Kurt. My childhood friends were such a strong link to all I had ever been or aspired to be. They were a reminder of my life during a time when life was simpler, before I lost all the instructions. They were especially dear. They knew who Diane Friel really was. They saw me (or so I fervently hoped) as I had been.

Some months after my visit to Washington, D.C., Kurt came to Florida to visit his brother and a friend, and spent a few days with my family. I was ecstatic. I tried to show him the "old Florida" as well as the new. We went to my beloved jetties at Ponce Inlet.

During the last day of Kurt's visit, another former classmate, Roy, now living in northern Florida, joined us. We dined at a favorite Greek restaurant, which featured belly dancing. It was the same restaurant in which I had danced years before.

As is the custom, the dancer requested members of the audience to join her on stage. Each of the others in the party took their turn. I did not want to get on stage with the young dancer, but at the urging of the others, did so. I had not given a thought to the fact that the leg positions of the belly dance could be maintained in the tight black sheath dress I was wearing.

The video they shot of the evening showed me in the most egregious display, akin to the bump and grind of a stripper, I had ever seen. I was greatly chagrined and embarrassed and immediately erased my performance from the video. Now, if only my former classmates had my memory problem, the incident could be totally erased. Somehow, I think they will probably remember my opprobrious conduct for the remainder of their lives. Life is not always kind.

My neurologist filed forms for my private disability

insurance policy and social security benefits. I panicked at the finality, and told my husband I was going to try to find something I could do.

"Like what?"

"I can't believe I am really out," I stammered. The speech pattern is often the last capacity to go, but I found I was unable to speak fast enough for Jack when in a rare discussion with him.

"Diane, stop humiliating yourself. It is time. You are beyond working any more. I insist. Listen to your doctor."

.   .   .

The electric bill was higher than usual because my clothes dryer was not shutting off automatically. I frequently forgot to remove the clothes from the dryer and there were many days when the laundry load tumble-dried all day. Jack was furious, emphasizing how much current the clothes dryer used. All I had to do was remember to take the clothes out, he said. But first, I thought, I have to remember that I put them in.

"Jack," I began hesitating slightly. "Today when I went to the doctor I passed someone in a wheelchair going into an office."

"So?"

"He was working. In a wheelchair."

"Look, Diane. He was a paraplegic. You have lost your mind. That is different."

"I haven't lost my mind! Don't say that!" I screamed

71

in defiance. "I have a neurological disability. It is my brain, Jack!"

He smiled at me smugly, sarcasm oiling his voice.

"Diane, where is your mind? Hm? Where is it located?"

I understood his wretched meaning, and could not find the words to refute his disparaging remark.

I retreated to my bedroom and idly began leafing through manuscripts I had written: fiction, non-fiction, humor, short stories, even mysteries. I had always enjoyed writing and had dreamed as a child of becoming a writer.

Both of my far away "little school friends" had recently encouraged me to continue trying. I picked up a blue manuscript, neatly bound: a chronicle of my battles with strokes, neurologists, and a declining vascular system over the years. I had done considerable research for its preparation. In disgust, I tossed it into the trash, then retrieved it and tore the pages out, one by one.

I had told my neurologist I was preparing the chronicle to aid future patients, perhaps my own descendants. He encouraged me and said he would like to read it, give his opinion. He said I should continue to write, whether good, bad or indifferent. It was an outlet, and a means of keeping my brain cells alive.

Perhaps he was right. I expected to begin saying, "Duh, duh, duh," any day, now.

Rummaging through the scattered manuscripts and

loose papers, I unexpectedly came across another copy of the manuscript I had just destroyed. It didn't want to go away. Perhaps something could be done with it after all. It might even benefit others some day.

Months passed, and I was staying alone in the darkened house. Only letters from my faraway friends broke my depression. I was becoming increasingly paranoid. My sensitivities were much too high. I required Jack's escort to the grocery due to my damaged inner compass. He would telephone during the day to remind me to do the laundry or other duties. Meals were haphazard. Jack chided me regularly because I frequently forgot to eat during the day.

I was approved for disability benefits. The day the approval came in the mail, my world exploded. I spent the entire afternoon sobbing, and trying to sort out what I should do now. Jack came home to find me distraught in the kitchen, trying to throw things about to vaguely resemble a meal. I was still fighting the miserable, uncontrolled sobbing. Jack, with all of his volatile moods, had not been able to reduce me to tears for a long time. He was startled to see them flowing so readily.

He sounded genuinely concerned as he asked me to tell him what had happened.

Jerkily, I told him I had been approved for benefits. He put his hand on my shoulder.

"Diane, that is good news," he said softly. "Why are you crying?"

"Because I thought they would say no! Don't you see?

This means it is really true, all of it! I want my records! I want to see. . . I want to see. . ."

Jack said we would get my updated records. We needed to have a file on this, anyway. He was becoming less volatile, less argumentative. He assured me he would take care of me. I could depend upon him.

When the long-awaited records arrived, I recoiled at the lab reports. Staring dumbly at them, I realized that I was looking at the clinical proof. It was not what someone had said. It was the results of my latest lab tests.

Silently, I put the records away in a medical file, and hid them along with the blank Living Will.

One day I stood in front of the enormous mirrored closet doors that covered   one entire wall of my bedroom. I studied my reflection closely. I looked perfect. I looked untouched. No one could tell just by looking at me that I wasn't perfect any more. Suddenly a spasm went through me. I clasped my hands tightly over my mouth to stifle the scream that was rising from my throat and trying to spill out into the quiet room. ❧

8

LAST CHANCE REUNION

I was grateful for Marie's personable letters. They helped me hang on when I felt there was nothing to hang onto. Initially Kurt had also been a great boon to my spirits. He gave me kindly advice and good wishes, but gradually wrote less and less.

One morning my mail contained a surprise letter from Roy, the former classmate who had joined us at the Greek restaurant during Kurt's visit. He was holding a mini-reunion at his beach house in northern Florida, and I was invited. Part of me thrilled to this, as I had never been invited to the large reunions of my former classmates. Another part of me recoiled in fear of my inferiority being discovered. Perhaps I would get lost, or behave inappropriately? What if the other attendees did not welcome me? What if they did not even remember me?

I telephoned Marie at her home in Ohio. She was not sure she could attend, but insisted that I should go and have "a great time." I knew I could not attend without some moral support. A lot of moral support.

Next I called Kurt, to determine if he was attending. Receiving no answer, I telephoned Roy, the host, and inquired if he had received an RSVP from Kurt. Roy advised me that Kurt would not be able to attend.

Marie called to say she could come and asked me to check on reservations at the motel nearest the scheduled reunion. I gleefully began to plan all the varied activities we would undertake once together after so many years. It was arranged that she would fly to Orlando and we would both drive up the coast to the gathering.

Shortly before Marie was due to arrive, I caved in to feelings of paranoia and insecurity, certain that I would not be really welcome, and would not be remembered by my former classmates. I canceled our motel reservations, and instead made reservations, paid in advance, for the beach at my favorite coastal haven near Ponce Inlet.

I was astonished by Marie's reaction. She stated emphatically that I was indeed attending, if she had to drag me all the way up Highway A-1-A. I reserved the canceled room at the site of the reunion once more. However, I did not cancel the Ponce Inlet reservation. Although I could not afford to have reservations at motels on two different parts of Florida's coast, I could not release my fail-safe key. If I was not greeted warmly, or did not feel comfortable at the reunion, I needed an escape hatch.

Marie was concerned over my paranoia and trepidation. Much as she tried to alleviate my insecurity, however, she could not.

As usual these days, I had mixed feelings. Part of me was very anxious to see as many of my former class-mates as possible. The next large reunion would be four years down the line, and judging by the rate of my decline, I would not be attending. But much as I wanted to attend, I was also terrified that the others would not welcome me.

I wrote letters of inquiry to two former classmates who had treated me kindly when we were children, to find out if they were attending. And I wrote Kurt, asking to please advise if he was not attending, as I then would most likely not, either. And hang Marie's objections. Then immediately prior to the date of the reunion, I received a note from Kurt. He would attend. I felt a wave of relief that at least I would have two friends there. That day I bought a gift for Kurt as a tribute for his many past kindnesses, and had it engraved with my sentiments.

Marie arrived for our get-together, and we drove up the coast to the reunion. Upon arriving, I was greeted warmly by two former classmates, Jim and Nancy Morrow. The two were friendly, excellent conversa-tionalists. Jim had suffered a bout of encephalitis a few years before, and was left with some minor but perma-nent memory loss. Still, he possessed a finely tuned sense of humor and kept me smiling at his witticisms. Perhaps it was the old adage that "it takes one to know one," or "misery loves company," but Jim greeted me most effusively and conversed more with me than any-one else attending.

His wife, Nancy, came in a close second, and we were both chatting during the afternoon, when the subject of short-term memory loss arose. Nancy stated that her husband suffered only a minor problem with short-term retention since his illness. I nonchalantly stated that I, also, had sustained some loss, but that I had acquired a technique of hiding it. Nancy gave me a qualm as she looked steadily into my eyes and quietly advised me otherwise.

"They can read you, Diane," she murmured. "They can. Believe me. They can read you."

I tried to talk with Kurt as I needed some of his wise advice. However, he behaved strangely, as though I had leprosy. The others, including the host, Roy, and his wife, whom I had entertained at the dinner party with Kurt, made me feel invisible. Either something was amiss or my paranoia was out of control.

One other attendee, a Don Juan playboy, acknowledged my presence with a ready flow of conversation. He had a line my mother could have hung an entire week's wash on, but I was grateful for conversation – even though it was svelte chatter.

After one day at the reunion, Marie noticed my reticence and told me she was ready to leave at any time and travel down the coast to New Smyrna's Ponce Inlet with me. We said farewell to the group, and I took the initiative and hugged curt Kurt as I left. I was fighting tears of regret as I gazed at my former classmates. We had known each other since first grade and I was looking at them for probably the very last time, ever.

As I descended the wooden stairs leading to where my car was parked, Jim Morrow asked if I would be attending their big reunion in four years. I turned and looked at him, not speaking, and he repeated the question, thinking I had not heard him.

Swallowing the lump in my throat, I whispered, "We'll see if I can be there." I rushed down the remaining steps and into my car before I began openly crying and embarrassing everyone.

Marie was puzzled by my certainty that I would never again see the group of acquaintances I had known since before we had permanent teeth. My emotions were raw and I reluctantly confided to Marie the reasons for it all, including a bout with paranoia. I divulged my fears about the future. She listened with profound interest, compassion and understanding.

Marie and I had a relaxing few days at the jetty beach, acting like two schoolgirls again. I laughed so much I lost my voice the second day there. I was the old Diane Friel again, if only for a while.

Shortly after the reunion, I sent a bottle of French perfume to Roy's wife as a hostess gift, and a postcard to each of the other attendees stating it had been good to see them after so many years. I sent Jim Morrow money and a request for copies of his photographs of the gathering, as my own left a lot to be desired.

Good-natured Jim complied with excellent shots of the group. I heard nothing from the hostess regarding the hostess gift, and heard nothing more from Kurt Fuller. He had not thanked me for his gift, either. I was now convinced beyond a doubt that either my conduct or conversation had given me away as being of diminished capacities. I was certain they had not liked me. My heart was aching.

Telling myself I had to become accustomed to such intellectual snobbery did no good. I knew them "when." And I knew Kurt Fuller well.

So I purchased a special photo album and placed the photographic memories of my D.C. trip, Kurt's visit, and the mini-reunion neatly inside, arranging each picture with care. A line from the screenplay "Inherit the Wind" came into my thoughts (a rare occurrence those days):

"The loneliest thing in the world is to be standing when everyone around you is sitting. . . and they all look at you and ask, 'What is wrong with her?'"

9

JEOPARDIZED RIGHTS

I still had not executed the Living Will tucked secretively away in my bedroom. I did, however, execute a Power of Attorney granting my husband authority to act on my behalf regarding a small personal investment I had made years ago. I filled out the document, had my signature guaranteed by our bank, and then carefully placed the Power of Attorney into my bank account folder. Should I deteriorate greatly, my husband would find the Power of Attorney when reviewing my statements.

I managed to cling to a small shred of independence by zealously keeping this information to myself. I feared that if I divulged the details of the small account, he would insist I empty it to pay off mounting bills. I had a few other small shreds of independence, as well.

In the kitchen I labored to provide well-balanced meals, although food and cooking utensils alike were

81

frequently charred beyond salvation. I put much care into meal preparation, keeping them simple, thereby giving myself at least an opportunity to succeed. Following recipes was chancey, at best. I clung to that part of my duties as though they were a life raft, pushing the day when I could no longer cook at all far off into the future. In fact, I preferred to believe that such a day would never arrive.

My housekeeping was minimal. When more extensive cleaning or refurbishing was required, I would push the projects aside, hoping for "a better day" when I would not feel so overwhelmed.

I cherished visits from my two young grandchildren, yet guiltily restricted them to short stays. This gave me a better chance to enjoy them without encountering problems. I feared having an incident when they were with me which would make their parents reluctant to permit visits at all. Out of necessity, I was visiting with them less often.

The most valuable tool of independence was my automobile, a small white convertible. I became a most rigorously defensive driver. Nothing must take this liberty from me. I worried that although I had my doctor's permission to continue driving, any infraction or fender bender would probably cost me my cherished license. I fretted that my driving days would be ended when my full medical condition was brought into the Florida sunlight.

I feared the possibility of someday losing control over my own home, my own meals, my own family, and my own automobile. In short, I feared losing my last shred of dignity and control over myself. My diagnosis exposed me to the elements. My rights had become tenuous and delicate. They existed only so long as nothing untoward occurred.

This rendered me helpless, stranded with my tender underbelly exposed to the vagaries of family and strangers alike.

"I mustn't get into any trouble or I will be forced to relinquish all of my human rights."

I still had not achieved the ability to live for today alone; the uncertain future did not allow for that. But I knew I must work at it. The bridge I was crossing was precarious enough due to its missing planks. I had to stop attempting to cross other bridges before I reached them. ☙

10

SEXUALITY

*T*here was one tender part of me that I needed to expose to someone. Highly sensual even when a very young woman, I had evolved into a woman with heightened sexual desires. My desires became a source of frustration for my husband, who, unfortunately, had reached a point of declining interest. Whether this decline was due to the simple advance of time, or to a physical ailment he chronically suffers, I did not know.

An increased sexual drive often develops as Alzheimer's Disease progresses. This is a vital and extremely frustrating problem for many people in the early to moderate stages. Despite all my difficulties, I now felt like Libido Lady.

I was equipped with a sex drive accelerating at the speed of a rocket but with nowhere to drive. Or, as a male might put it, "The problem is not with the lead in my pencil. I just have no one to write to!"

Increased tension developed between my spouse and I as we each tried to cope with this new development. He was struggling with a tender ego, and I had to be cautious not to affront such a delicate attribute as a male ego. Heaven forbid!

I desired, and physically and emotionally needed warm, passionate touch; to feel my body acquiesce and spasmodically explode in return. I could not remember the last time I saw the look of true arousal in a man's eyes.

Meanwhile, I was reaching the point where even commercials for water massagers or the more sensual commercials for perfumes or wines caught my interest. I wondered why men were so easily controlled during sex, but so uncontrollable with their pants on.

I approached my specialists and general practitioner with my embarrassing problem and timidly requested a prescription to lessen my libido. My requests were denied. My general practitioner even laughed uncontrollably, asking if I realized that what I considered a problem, the rest of the world would consider a great asset.

It was during a trip with a friend — a Professor Emeritus who has been forced to relinquish his long tenure with a large University due to early-onset Alzheimer's — that I too laughed heartily at the predicaments of my libido life. At our favorite beach, the professor drank a very small bottle of wine, and tossed the empty bottle onto the backseat of my convertible. After delivering him safely home and returning to mine, I discovered his empty wine bottle in my car — lying on his discarded socks and underwear briefs! Evidently he had placed his underwear on my back seat after changing his clothes, and forgot to retrieve them. (We have this "little memory problem.")

I stared for a moment in confusion at the wine bottle and underwear scattered on the car seat. Then a wave of laughter shook me as I envisioned the predicament if my husband, instead of me, had discovered the array. He might have thought I'd found another means of alleviating "Alzheimer's Libido."

I washed my fellow traveler's undergarments and mailed them with a note, "Miss anything yet?"

• • •

I finally threw away one of my last vestiges of propriety and attempted the "do it yourself" method — masturbation. But I didn't know how. Perplexed, I dissuaded myself by admonishing that probably the church, and certainly my mother, would not have approved. Women didn't do that. Men did that.

My outgoing, mercurial, joking nature to the contrary, I have always been rather chaste regarding sex and reluctant to self-indulge. When you are a 1937 model born of an extremely uptight Puritanical family, you do not dare broadcast that you greatly enjoy sex with a partner, much less explore the solitaire scenario.

Finally I swallowed my last ounce of pride and inquired of a greatly trusted friend "how to." My friend appeared more shocked by the fact that I did not know how, than by the query, itself. The trusted confidante referred me to a book on female sexuality which would explain "the mechanics in detail."

Mechanics were indeed what this sex goddess needed — or electronics, to be explicit. To achieve sexual relief, I resorted to using a vibrator.

Although it had taken a great deal of courage to approach my dear friend with the initial query, it took much more to attempt to "do-it-myself." I locked all doors, closed all draperies, hid all electronic evidence, and in truth, do not believe I could have been more secretive and discreet if I had a lover in the house.

I have shared this most vulnerable part of my coping simply because you, also, may be in the "need to know" legion.

As I march — or am dragged — further into Alzheimer's Disease, I am less ashamed of my more primal urges. Consequently, I am also far less judgmental of others for theirs. Perhaps it is a result of premature dementia, but I think not. It is more likely the realization that I am probably coming toward my final stretch — that I have experienced many "last times" without understanding they were, indeed, the last time.

This knowledge enables me to savor life more openly and ravenously. I appreciate all good things more, whether they be trusted friends, cherished memories, nature's beauty — or physical pleasures. ❧

11

DUTIES

*T*ax time came around. Time for gathering documents and receipts and conferring with our accountant. This had always been my responsibility as my background and training involved meticulous recordkeeping. This year, my husband Jack expected me to carry on as before and provide our accountant with the necessary data. I was stunned when I realized he did not intend to take over this very important annual responsibility.

For most of one entire day, I sat surrounded by scribbled notes, torn receipts, and proofs of income earned and lost. Finally, I realized I was mentally mired in quicksand, and just gathered all of the documentation into a large pocketed folder.

I set out for the tax accountant's office with plenty of time to spare, in case I should take a wrong turn or become lost. As I pulled neatly into an available parking place, I breathed a deep sigh of relief. Leaning back against the headrest, I paused a moment to gather my wits. Reaching out for the folder, I was chagrined to realize it was not there. I had driven to the appointment without one single tax document.

Quickly I restarted the engine and began my journey home to retrieve the folder. By the time I reached my home I was frustrated, and ran throughout the house looking for the folder. Finally locating it, I ran back to my car. My throat was dry and tight, but I did not feel I could take the time to get a drink of water.

Arriving at the accountant's office quite late, I waited in his outer office while he finished other duties which had arisen in the meantime. Laboriously, he sorted through my clumsy notes and receipts. He had been told of my diagnosis, and expressed his kind sympathy, adding that my disorder was "something we associate with people in their seventies or eighties, not at your age, Diane."

I hesitantly tried to explain to our tax wizard that the term, "premature" did, indeed, infer ahead of schedule — atypical.

Perhaps I was now into another phase of acceptance. For the first time I was explaining to someone else the frustrations of being a comparatively young, early onset, early diagnosed victim, instead of someone explaining it to me. I had also associated all of the dementias, not just Alzheimer's, with the elderly, and that made it harder to accept my lot. I was not elderly. I was not totally incognizant, incontinent or incompetent.

Our accountant was usually able to give me an educated guess as to how much we would owe in income taxes. Now due to the haphazard documentation, he would have to work on our return for a few days before giving us his assessment. He also suggested my husband and I consult with an attorney regarding legal documents we may require in the future, and to explore "alternatives." I stared at him in confusion. What alternatives?

Later that evening, I told my husband of the accountant's suggestion that we consult an attorney. My spouse sighed, then said that we could put that off for a while, since I had been stabilized for a few months at this same plateau.

"If and when you start to worsen again, we can see an attorney at that time," he added.

One week later I received a call from the accountant's office. We were to receive a sizable refund, instead of owing a significant amount as I had feared. I was certain a mistake had been made. The poor clerk at the other end of the telephone painstakingly went over each entry of the form, and I pretended to understand them all. I didn't. My husband returned from work as I was finishing the call, and I told him that there must be some mistake, urging him to go to the accountant and examine every detail thoroughly. I could not put my mind at rest and accept our good news. It was fixed in my mind that we were going to owe thousands of dollars, and nothing could exorcise my fixation on doom and gloom.

Upon his return home from the accountant, my elated spouse attempted to go over the form with me. It was pointless. Finally, he instructed me to sign it on the designated line beneath his signature and mailed the confusing form to the big tax office in the sky.

He agreed that from that date on, he would be responsible for all of our tax matters and the keeping of records. I doubted his efficiency in that regard, but crossed my fingers. Beggars cannot be choosers.

Simple addition and subtraction, such as is necessary for keeping a balanced checkbook, was no longer possible for me. I required a large-keyed calculator for the most perfunctory entries. The bank statement seldom now agreed with our checkbook balance, so I developed a habit of keeping one hundred dollars "hidden" in the checking account, i.e., not entered in the book and thereby becoming at least a one hundred dollar cushion for my errors. Occasionally my husband would write a billfold check without entering it into our book, and I pounced on this oversight as though totally responsible for the never-balancing checkbook.

Both of my sons again contacted me this year with questions regarding their own tax matters. I was aghast. Did they realize I was no longer playing with a full deck, or not? One moment they behaved as though I was at risk whenever out and about alone. The next moment they were asking my opinions on complicated tax matters.

I did not know the answers. I did not even understand the questions.

Routinely I drive two blocks to a fast food restaurant accompanied by my little white mixed terrier, Scampi. We drive through the carry out line and order two biscuits. The employees at the restaurant are always cheerful, and speak to Scampi and I as we pick up our treat. One day I was returning alone from an errand

91

and decided to stop by for the biscuits en route. Surprisingly, the manager ran out of the restaurant, asking in a worried tone, "What happened to your little white dog?"

I advised him that Scampi was busy and had sent me after his biscuit.

On another occasion, as I pulled up to the speaker to give my order, Scampi barked sharply before I could say a word. A laughing voice acknowledged him with a simple, "Please drive through."

"You are late today," she advised as we passed through.

I drove away smiling in spite of myself. My life had become so very predictable! Was this pathetic, or what? ⌒⌐

12

OPPOSITE ENDS OF THE TELESCOPE

*M*y husband continued to believe that everything will work out to my eventual salvation; I also clung to that belief and was nurtured by it. My brother preferred to put on a blindfold, hoping that what he did not have to actually hear or see did not exist. He became more detached, and most of our conversations were by telephone although he resided only ten miles away.

I protected my ailing father from full knowledge of my diagnosis and prognosis. He was aware I had a spatial problem and no longer had an inner compass to guide me, but appeared to believe that I was no longer working because my husband had decided to give his wife a life of leisure.

My elder son Bill preferred to ignore the entire subject of my difficulties. One day when he was visiting, I called him into the kitchen to ascertain whether I had turned on the correct burner of my twenty-two year old stove. Although I had cooked on that range for two decades, I could not figure which knob controlled which burner, nor where the varying degree positions were located.

"Oh, good grief, I don't believe this!" he exclaimed.

Later, I purchased a new stove which has the markings clearly imprinted, and the location of each burner shown on small diagrams above each knob.

Once I tried to explain to Bill that I was having a deuce of a time going anywhere due to becoming forever lost. He quipped, "I don't understand that, Mom; you always find the male go-go dancers." He was wittily referring to the previous summer when I took two women friends of many years to an establishment in our area featuring such beefcake.

My daughter was always quick to laugh, and just as quick to explode in anger. She inherited my propensity to worry. Worrying is what Lynn and I do best, much to the disgust of our laid-back spouses. However, as she matured, I saw in her a tendency to hold herself detached from problems whenever expedient for her. Whether self-serving or self-protecting, only her inner self and God can know. There is a difference.

My youngest, Shaun, aged twenty-one, was the most supportive and protective. Although he was partially in denial of my situation, it was evident that Shaun did, indeed realize my predicament. He would canvass the house whenever he came over to visit, discarding expired milk and other foodstuffs from the refrigerator. Sometimes he would demand to know if I had eaten "any of this stuff" lately, and he would caution me regarding my general health. On another occasion when I had not been at an appointed place at the designated time, he and his sister drove through an entire section of town searching for me. Shaun was livid with worry.

Though Shaun repeatedly told me to cease worrying about my wretched diagnosis, I was "doing fine, just fine." it was this same heir to my throne who panicked when I walked home from a medical appointment instead of awaiting my scheduled pick-up. I can still see the amazed look on his face when, after an hour of fruitless search he drove home to alert his father (and probably the local gendarmes) of my disappearance, only to find me safely at home after my long and thoughtless walk.

"I can't believe you made it," he murmured, staring in wonder at his now unpredictable mother. "I really can't. I am totally surprised, Mom. And don't ever do it again."

Shaun also frequently urged me in conversation to "speed it up, Mom, speed it up." This only made things worse and I would stammer nervously. I was "already dancing as fast as I could."

Early one morning I entered my bathroom accompanied by my faithful white terrier, Scampi, and discovered a large hairy rodent perched on the commode seat. Scampi and I stumbled over each other beating a confused retreat. Outside the door, I thought, "No! Even New York does not have rats that big!" I reopened the door partially and saw an opossum had apparently entered our pet door and climbed up to the commode seat. I telephoned Shaun and requested he come over and evict the 'possum in the privy.

"Mom, what is a 'possum doing in your bathroom?" he asked incredulously.

"Sitting on the commode," I truthfully answered.

Shaun's voice was syrupy calm and sweet as he instructed me to sit down, stay calm, and do nothing, absolutely nothing, until he arrived. I could tell he did not believe I had a beast in the bathroom. When he arrived, he had his longtime girlfriend with him. They each took up station next to me, inquiring as to my health. I asked wasn't he going to get rid of that 'possum?

Shaun sighed, then agreed to look into my bathroom. After one split second, he turned, and in a disbelieving voice whispered to his girlfriend, "There really is a 'possum in there!"

The 'possum in the privy was quickly removed to the back yard and my flagging acuity was vindicated.

Sometime after, while updating my daughter Lynn during a visit, Shaun advised confidentially, "It's like this. Most of the time Mom has to give everything a second thought to understand it. The remainder of the time she simply forgets it altogether."

Lynn had the most stoic attitude of my children. A distance of two thousand miles between us obviously helped. In our long-distance conversations she would repeatedly tell me to "slow down, slow down, you're talking ninety miles an hour, Mom. I am only understanding part of what you are saying!"

Obeying my younger son's request to "speed it up" so

that Lynn would not determine any additional deterioration often backfired.

My two grandchildren, aged eleven and four, were the most forthright, as is usually the case with children. At one time I had frequently taken them to the local park, the beach, circus, or to movies and fast food restaurants. That was now over. What was, was. The children quickly understood that I was diminishing in capacities, without being told. They began "taking care" of me, instead of vice versa. When I tired or became churlish quickly, they began asking the repeated and revealing questions, "Are we making you nervous? Is something wrong?"

The worst scenario took place one day when they came to visit, and I actually forgot they were in my home, and retired to my room for a nap, leaving them to their own devices. The four-year-old is not the type of child one leaves to his own devices — ever.

After months of confused introspection about my plight and my family's apparent stoicism, the fact finally dawned on me that we were viewing my condition from opposite positions. It was as though I was standing at one end of a telescope and my family at the other, each peering intently into the instrument, each with a quite opposite perspective.

I recoiled in alarm at each additional loss of memory, and concentration. But I would not confide in family members as each additional loss occurred. Instead I continued playing a camouflage game of "I've Got A Secret," long after everyone knew. Each loss was magnified in my fear and grief, yet I continued my foolish attempt at deception.

From the opposite end of the telescope, my family focused not on what was now missing, but on what remained. I realized part of this was their own form of denial. However, through Shaun (who was more outspoken and protective than my elder offspring), I also realized that my beloved family was aligned at the other end of my life's telescope.

I arrived at the conclusion that they were probably on the right track. They were observing me, but concentrating on what I still had and not on what I had lost. My family was standing at the correct end of the telescope, while I was peering at the situation from the wrong end, and viewing a more distorted image.

My husband had ceased beginning discussions with the words, "Do you remember. . ." and now talked to me about experiences we had shared as though advising me for the first time. Indeed, sometimes his reminiscences were lost from my memory. Other times, however, his words would spark a memory still alive and retrievable within my brain, giving me a chance to expand, "Yes, and that was also when. . ." It was a kind way of determining whether I had recall of that particular occurrence, without humiliation. Asking if I could remember a particular event was demeaning, regardless of whether I could remember it or not. I felt much more comfortable when he simply recounted an event, as it left the door open for me to either listen to this "new" old memory or to join in his remembrance.

Resolve swept through me. I was experiencing a mental breakthrough! From now on, I must concentrate on what I have, not what I have lost. ᴄ▲ᴇ

13

EBBING SAND IN THE HOURGLASS

I had many unfounded fears and became obsessively preoccupied by troubling stories in the media. At the same time, I displayed unwise disregard for my own safety (such as the incident of walking home from my medical appointment). I would frequently race throughout the house in a desperate search for my "missing" spouse, only to find him busy in his workshop or working in the yard.

My husband sometimes had a most confusing and frustrating attitude. He would instruct me to perform errands that taxed my waning capacities, and developed the hurtful habit of gesturing in the "wrap it up" hand movement whenever I tried to speak to him at length. At the sight of that wretched hand sign, my speech would immediately falter and I would begin stammering, losing my train of thought altogether.

He pressed me beyond my capabilities, yet frequently telephoned home during his workday to ask how I was.

He could know by simply looking at me upon his return home if I had a good day or a bad one. I attempted to hide the bad days from him as another pointless attempt at "I've Got a Secret." Unfortunately I never knew how he could diagnose the good day or bad day, so I wasn't certain how my performance should go. I gradually gave up on that deception, as I did not have the concentration to deceive him after a bad day.

Late-night restlessness and insomnia became vicious ogres. Once sleep finally came, it was a restless sleep with volatile and troubling dreams. My weight dropped dramatically. I was previously touted by my peers as "one of the lucky ones," in that my measurements remained the same as when I was a young woman. The weight loss rendered me emaciated. I put great effort into gaining weight, and after a year of trying, I finally regained eight of the lost pounds, improving my appearance.

My behavior was often repetitive as I checked and rechecked the date, the time of day, the location of my purse and other belongings. I was rapidly developing fetishes or mannerisms indicative of slipping capacities. I would ask my husband the date repeatedly. My language became saltier. I ceased driving at night or out of my immediate neighborhood, yet became anxious and frantic when I was a passenger as someone else drove. However, my laundry might remain in the washer or dryer for an inordinate period of time, usually until discovered by my husband.

I experienced an intense need for tender attention, loyalty, and affection. Yet I was reluctant to develop new friendships. I became cautious about conversing with telephone or door-to-door salespersons in case I might be unfairly persuaded to purchase a costly and unneeded item.

I continued my efforts to stop smoking. I tried every method on the market and invented some of my own. I was well aware of the effects of nicotine on the brain and wanted to give my cerebral functions a fair shake. A brain already struggling does not need the added detriment of toxins pumped into it. I also wanted to stop before I became a fire hazard. It could happen.

I had studied classical piano for several years in my youth and had even aspired to become a classical pianist. As an adult, my piano had become my tranquilizing therapy and also a much enjoyed hobby. Now I discovered I could no longer read music easily, my playing had become quite wooden, and I was dismayed that I sometimes could not recall the names of favorite pieces and their composers. I tried moving my musical hobby into the popular and country field, but it was of no use. My ability had all but vanished. All I retained was an immense joy in listening to recorded music. I enjoyed most of all the recordings of my youth and the simpler, heartfelt renditions of country performers. I could not abide the strident modern hard rock of today.

Guilt arose as a hounding enemy as I avoided situations wherein I was doomed to fail. My father became seriously ill, and underwent his second quad by-pass surgery. I forced myself to be present in the hospital on the day of his surgery. Once he had been moved to progressive care, however, I feigned reasons for not visiting him in the labyrinth of corridors and floors of the large medical facility. During my two days there, I experienced a soul searing confrontation with my deficits.

Becoming hopelessly lost, I finally whispered to a kind-looking nurse that I was an Alzheimer's patient, and requested she give me simply-drawn directions to the waiting room. She wrote down the directions and then escorted me to the elevator.

As I entered the elevator with many others, I noticed a distinguished man in a navy blue suit board the elevator beside me. As he entered, he somehow deleted all the other floor destinations and, much to my relief, he pushed the button to my floor. As we exited, he asked to see the room number and directions the nurse had placed into my perspiring palm. I was astounded. How did he know I had such instructions? After reading the note tightly gripped in my fist, he escorted me to a nurse's station, and asked the staff to assist me. I do not know who this man was, but suspect he was a physician who had overheard me whisper to the directing nurse.

Such individuals are the unsung but much appreciated saviors of the Alzheimer's patient. ☜☞

14

FEARS

*M*y most troublesome fears revolved around the same theme. Would my husband of over twenty years protect and take care of me should I decline further? He is a stalwart, a stoic, and we had only recently regained a state of grace in our marriage, after many troubled years. What if he should tire of a wife without her senses about her, should that be my future?

What would become of me? I needed his moral support and repeatedly sought his vow to take care of me for the rest of my life. Upon receiving his assurance once again, I would then inquire if he knew just how difficult keeping it may become in the future. It was as though I was trying to challenge his vow, to shake his resolve with every frightening detail of what might happen if I continued to deteriorate. I desperately needed reassurance. For the most part he quietly reaffirmed that he would take care of me forever, and that should my needs ever become such that he could

not handle them, he would simply cross that bridge
when he came to it, one step at a time.

To terminate this type of pointless exchange, he usually insisted that I would never deteriorate to the point
of totally losing myself. He knew my objective: to hang
in and hang tough until medical breakthroughs provide me with a means to cease my downhill slide.

Another fear raised its gargoyle features when my husband was diagnosed with a chronic and incurable kid-
ney ailment. Due to elevated blood pressure and cho-
lesterol, he was also at risk for a heart attack. I worried that should he require my care, could I provide
it? Probably not, I realized.

Upon the heels of that new fear followed the realization that if my husband should become incapacitated
or die, I would be alone. Like most wives, I could not
contemplate the possibility of losing my spouse of
twenty-five years. My concern, however, was com-
pounded by the uncertainty of my own medical future.

Not only that, but fear was also piercing my heart with
the knowledge that Alzheimer's is a familial, obviously
genetic neurological disorder. As such, I may have
unknowingly bequeathed it to my children — even
grandchildren — this wretched legacy which was just
as innocently inherited by me.

There is an old saying, "When children are young,
they step on your toes; when grown, they step on your
heart." Although I had three grown children, the very
thought of becoming a burden to any one or all of
them appalled me. Additionally, of course, I had the
attitude of most mothers, that should I need to fall
upon any of my children's care, God help me.

Although adults, they still appeared as children to me. Children, not caregivers.

What would become of me should my condition deteriorate? Would I be cared for, treated with kindness and concern? Or would I be an unwelcome and resented burden, a source of contention? Or worse, deemed non-existent? Would I be permitted to retain any degree of dignity and quality of life? Or would I be considered human refuse, without merit, without feelings?

I could well understand the desperation of those with serious illnesses who had ended their lives out of fear and uncertainty about the future. As the news announced the indictment of a Michigan physician who had assisted terminally ill individuals to commit suicide, I listened in despair. Despite all my fears about the future, I could not consider suicide as an option.

Nonetheless, I felt it should be a matter of choice for those living with chronic illnesses. The choice to float gently from this life as opposed to becoming a forced victim of pain should be theirs. Whenever I got on my soapbox about this moral minefield, others gazed at me in all too revealing concern. Let them think what they want, I sighed.

We are guaranteed the right to live, not the right to die. We are guaranteed only the pursuit of happiness, not its achievement. There are associations to prevent the prolonging of an animal's suffering, but our charitable kindness to pets does not extend to our fellow beings. Instead, a multitude of legal and religious barriers raise their heads, howling in outrage.
I knew what my pastor would say if he could hear my

philosophy. His voice would be low-key but firm in its
indictment of such a thought. Christian and Jewish
martyrs would be held before me by this man of the
cloth as an example. I do not know if I am of the
caliber of a martyr.

15

COUNSELING

I went through a cycle of spin-off depression and anxiety such as I had never before experienced. All of the patients I had seen or heard about were much worse than I. Surely this had to be some horrendous mistake! I eventually sought counseling again. I had to get out of that darkened room, somehow.

The doctor in charge confided to me that his father had suffered from Alzheimer's. He told me that while his father experienced similar symptoms, he had, never, "totally lost himself." He had his limitations but was able to function, still "himself." I was greatly encouraged and comforted by this knowledge.

The kind practitioner also advised me that a new drug, which had proven quite effective in research testing, was presently awaiting approval by the Federal Drug Administration. He encouraged me to continue writing, even though I now felt too diminished to have worthwhile thoughts. The doctor also said that he would like to read through my old manuscript describing my initial struggle with dementia.

My therapist was a female psychologist who had witnessed her husband's father struggle with Alzheimer's and she also encouraged me greatly.

As some of my fears and problems were due to marital tensions, my husband was encouraged to attend counseling sessions with me. My increased sexual drive was a source of great frustration. As my husband and I each endeavor to improve our marriage, my sexual frustration might diminish. Methods for coping were suggested to me, and I felt I saw a light at the end of the tunnel. I hoped it was not a train.

Gradually, in fractions not inches, I began to feel more at ease and in command. I felt more optimistic and my attitude improved, although I was still prone to tidal waves of fear and apprehension, coupled with despair at any disappointments. I learned to take my memory slips in stride.

One day I was attempting to get my youngest child's attention. I called to him, naming different family members and friends, even the family dog, as I struggled to remember his name. I knew he was my son, my baby — just could not remember what in blazes his name was!

Realizing that my murmuring of different names was intended for him, he turned and looked at me intently, then in a low, smooth, voice, said, "Mom, I am Shaun. Remember, Mom? Shaun!"

"Of course you are!" I exclaimed brightly, leaning forward to kiss him lightly on the cheek. "And don't you ever change, either!" ❧

16

REMINISCENCES

As my grip upon the present slips, more and more comfort is found within my memories of the past. Childhood nostalgia is so keen I can actually smell the aroma of the small town library where I spent so many childhood hours. A mixture of hardwood floors, marble, ancient bookshelves and the musty odor of old books, all gave the old building a peaceful, tranquilizing quiet akin to a church.

Although I have not seen snowflakes for decades, I can taste them on my tongue (as well as icicles — the forerunner to popsicles — plucked for sucking). I can experience the total, absolute quiet of a snowbound world. Even the bitter pain endured when warming my frozen fingers after walking to my piano teacher's home becomes a bittersweet memory. It was while warming my hands one afternoon that I watched the first televised coronation, that of Queen Elizabeth II. My piano teacher had moved her television to the foyer so that waiting and thawing students could observe the lengthy ceremony.

Visions of the first daffodils of an Ohio spring float through my memory. I recall their hesitant breaking through the still half-frozen Ohio soil and their pausing as though to check the above-ground temperature before bursting forth in their golden glory.

My own voice echoes in my ears as I remember laughing with great glee while chasing fireflies, or lightning bugs, across our front lawn on summer nights. I would capture some and place them in a covered glass jar, then sit in wonder at my twinkling "lantern."

I remember with fondness being taught to walk the railroad rails by my teen-aged aunts. I was always afraid of heights, so they bolstered me until I was able to conquer the fear sufficiently to walk the rail over a small trestle not far from my paternal grandmother's home. I remember the sound of the train whistle and the chugging of the steam engine cutting through the silent night as I lay comfortably in my grandmother's deep soft feather bed.

I remember my grandmother and her violin. As a very young girl she had graduated from a local college of music and subsequently played in a string ensemble until her young husband's accidental death which left her a widow with an infant. Her violin become only her hobby, albeit a much beloved one, as a result. The Christmas shortly before her death she had been covertly observed by one of my cousins, pulling herself from her sickbed, and standing erect before a large mirror. She placed her precious violin (which by now had lost some strings) beneath her chin and slowly, reverently, played, "Silent Night" on one string. Today I have that still beautiful instrument, complete with her diploma. I wonder what will become of such ancestral ties after I am gone.

In an effort to tie the past to the present, I put intense effort into keeping old friendships alive, and renewing old friendships dating back to my elementary school days. My dear friend, Marie Thomerson, aids me in this resolve, although at first she believed me simply gripped by a soul searing bout of nostalgia.

Sometimes my attempts to rekindle old relationships were pitiful and self-demeaning. I was desperate. These individuals knew the old Diane Friel, and through them I could lift the veil of time and view her, myself, once again. I liked what I saw!

I was and am inordinately appreciative of each and every kindness afforded me by friends and acquaintances, alike. I realize that everything we do, does indeed matter. There is no substitute for graciousness, no excuse for rudeness nor churlish behavior.

Although, or perhaps because I was so very intent on keeping flames of old friendships burning, I was dismally unsuccessful in many of those attempts. Some friends however, without being privy to the fact that I was undergoing any trauma or transformation, did indeed stand once again beside me in friendship and understanding.

For those who would not, or just could not adjust to painful changes I was undergoing, I understand!

They shall be missed. ᴆᴇ

17

THROUGH THE LABYRINTH

*O*n good days I am filled with hope and determination to maintain my present plateau until the arrival of a medical breakthrough. On bad days I realize I have about the same chance in this as winning Florida's lottery: one in about 15 million.

It is then that I have the worst sense of aloneness and lack of worth. Each one of us must feel they have worth as a living being — a person with the same rights and privileges as the people next door. I feel my lack of worth acutely when I am in large groups of people. Being in a crowd or even in a busy thoroughfare overwhelms me. All those people "of worth," with places to go — who know where they are going.

Painfully lonely, I still contrarily, deliberately, sit alone in my home. The radio and TV are silent. I am suspended. Somewhere there is that ever-present reminder list of what I am supposed to do today. But I cannot find it.

I decide to attempt to do the laundry and find myself
outside, in my backyard, holding soiled clothes. How
did I get here? How do I get back? I find my way
again, and also find wet clothing in the washer, dried
and wrinkled clothes in the dryer. How long have they
been there?

My husband telephones to determine my status. I try
to con him and terminate the call as quickly as possible. However, he discerns from my speech pattern that
this is a Bad Day, and advises me to stay put, go
nowhere (fat chance!) and do nothing until he
returns home. He inquires if I have eaten today. I
cannot remember, but answer affirmatively.

He inquires, "What did you eat?" Savvy wretch! I cannot even continue my attempt at deception now.
Tears begin to flow without warning and I am angry at
myself for their presence. He repeats his "stay put"
instructions and the call is finally terminated.

Another telephone call, this time from some lively
individual whom I cannot place, but who obviously
knows me well. I say I must hang up and return the
call later. I leave all future calls to my answering
machine and return to my solitude. I do not answer
the door bell.

I know there will always be periods when my lack of
worth gnaws at me, obstinately. However, I must hang
in and hang tough. My first efforts to find a publisher
for this manuscript were met with the response that
"Alzheimer's disease is a topic of too limited interest."
Too limited interest? With millions affected? With
such a high profile, today? Too limited interest.
Always a person of passion, I do not intend to take this
disorder with cold stoicism.

If I am no longer a woman, why do I still feel I'm one?
If no longer worth holding, why do I crave it? If no
longer sensual, why do I still enjoy the soft texture of
satin and silk against my skin? If no longer sensitive,
why do moving song lyrics strike a responsive chord in
me? My every molecule seems to scream out that I do,
indeed, exist, and that existence must be valued by
someone!

Without someone to walk this labyrinth by my side,
without the touch of a fellow traveler who truly under-
stands my need of self-worth, how can I endure the
rest of this uncharted journey? I thirst today for
understanding, a tender touch and healing laughter.

To help myself by helping others, I have started a support group for other early-diagnosed Alzheimer
patients — with sponsorship from the Alzheimer's
Association. I found I was not the only early diagnosed, early-onset victim in Orlando much in need of
mutual support. No matter how caring our friends
and family members are, we STILL NEED EACH
OTHER — people walking through the same maze as
ourselves. There were already support groups for
caregivers, but until now, nothing for us. "We, the
People."

My professor friend and fellow traveler gives me much-
needed support and encouragement. It is an "inside
joke" between us that we resent suffering from an ailment which sounds more like a beer than a disease.
In fact, he threatens to create a T-shirt emblazoned:
"Hello, I'm The Alzheimer Man!" We feel we deserve
better.

In a very casual manner, while sipping coffee one day,

another fellow traveler stated that we need to accept without grief the fact that Alzheimer's is a terminal disease.

I stared in shock. Misunderstanding my expression, my fellow traveler insisted that we must entertain no grief for our (again) "terminal situation." I objected, stating flatly that I did not ever consider myself terminally ill. Some of us reach plateaus where we hold for years, until we eventually, being mere mortals, expire of some other ailment unrelated to premature dementia.

"That's the girl!" my fellow traveler exclaimed with bravado.

"I'm not being brave!" I insisted. "In truth, I do not consider myself ill with a terminal condition, nor you! I consider us coping with a chronic, and," my voice cracked, "possibly a progressive one."

"Possibly?"

"It is not written in stone!" I exclaimed. "It does not have to be! 'It ain't necessarily so!'"

Sharing perspectives, fears, empathy, moral support — even a few healing laughs — is invaluable. Other people, those not in the labyrinth with us, may not understand our plight. Because we "look okay," others are surprised when we become lost in familiar surroundings. Because we "look okay," people raise an eyebrow when we cannot recall our children's ages, or perhaps their names. Because we "look okay," clerks become annoyed as we fumble, trying to count out the money for a purchase. Because we "look okay," some exchange curious glances when we insert an inappropriate or newly invented word into a sentence.

Despite my fears and uncertainties about the future, I seem to have conducted myself appropriately thus far. I have recently been credited with the attributes of "great courage," and of being "an incredible lady." One stranger even wrote me in capital letters that I was "ONE GUTSY LADY!" I do not feel courageous, much less gutsy. As for the acclaim that I am an "incredible lady," I do not know if the accent was on "incredible" or "lady." In any event, I feel unworthy of such praise. Mostly I feel insecure, confused, frightened and as though I am dancing as fast as I can.

But I still have my loved ones. I still have a home. I still have my private enjoyments which make life worthwhile. And although there are many days when I am painfully aware that less of me exists than the day before, for now, I can say, I am still here!

Diane McGowin exists! Perhaps someday, someone will be glad I did.

I am very blessed. ⌒⌐

EPILOGUE

BY DIANA MCGOWIN & JACK MCGOWIN

s my capacities dwindled over time, the word processor became a chief outlet. Speech sometimes faltered as my train of thought traveled too fast for the tongue, and on too many tracks simultaneously. The word processor had an unfailing memory, was adept at spelling, and could help me keep track of what I was writing about. The original manuscript for this book was stored on the faithful word processor; others assisted in refining and editing it when necessary.

An inanimate personal companion, however useful, has its limitations. Nothing can replace the value of a friend with whom the patient can relate. A good friend helps reduce pressure on the family to provide never-ending solace and understanding.

Despite a strident denial eating away deep inside me, I contacted various local organizations to locate a support group for "people like me." To my dismay, I found none. The reason is primarily because early-

117

diagnosed individuals usually don't contact such organizations for assistance; their care givers eventually make the initial contact, after the patient has deteriorated substantially. Evidently, no one had anticipated the need of patients who are still in the early to moderate stages, and may, indeed, **never** deteriorate to the incompetent state of the more severely incapacitated.

I began my effort to develop a support group for early-diagnosed victims. The local chapter of the Alzheimer's Association was most co-operative, encouraging and supportive. They invited me to speak before their Board meeting. A unanimous vote was registered, approving their sponsorship of the support group.

My husband Jack also attended the Board meeting, since he was required to drive me. It was as a result of this meeting that I heard Jack declare for the first time that he was proud of me. When the chairman lauded me for courage, I turned in surprise and confusion to my husband, who was silently nodding in agreement.

"Do you think I have courage?" I asked.

"Yes," he answered.

I do not feel courageous. I feel I am a pebble in a rapid brook. I hope this little pebble can send out ripples upon ripples, in an ever widening circle, until the ripples eventually lap up on a shore where someone like me is stranded and feeling alone.

The purpose of the support group is not to counsel or treat, but for us to have someone with whom we can relate, someone walking the same bridge we are walking. Bridge walking is hazardous when there are planks missing and the traveler must step with caution. Therefore, I stand with other patients, "people like me," requesting and giving moral support as we await a medical breakthrough. Support groups play a vital part in helping the patient maintain dignity and may even help slow down the loss of capacity. Certainly, the shared tears, laughter and hope are a balm to the troubled spirit.

As with any ailment, the patient has good days and bad days, and so, therefore, does the family. The patient's need for assistance and moral support increases as time goes by. It is at this stage that a pet is a great boon to the patient. Always loyal and loving, never critical but ever approving, a pet brings unconditional love. I have a much beloved and loving mixed terrier forever at my side, and a feisty Jardine parrot with whom I converse lightheartedly when alone. Other family members help me keep my pet friends clean and well fed.

Many patients never deteriorate to the invalid state. The reasons why one may be severely and rapidly afflicted while another deteriorates less and much more slowly is still being explored by researchers. At present, my capacities do not appear to be deteriorating as rapidly as they did initially. I seem to have reached a plateau where I am for the moment, holding firm. I am praying that I maintain a slower decline, and that researchers will soon develop a miracle aid for victims of this wretched ailment.

I have volunteered to participate in experimental drug testing and study programs, but to date have not been selected. My first request to take part in a volunteer research program was denied for vagaries of the test rules, but I am on a list for future research. A dear friend has cautioned me against participating in such research programs, especially those testing new drugs. However, I **must** participate; any improvements gained can only aid other victims in the future.

My husband supports my efforts, understanding my need for a degree of initiative and independence. He has always been strong; I hope he is Herculean as my dependency increases. He joins me in this hope.

I am taking vitamins from Sweden in an effort at tissue rejuvenation and perhaps the slowing of my loss. The vitamins are merely another example of ceaseless efforts and straw grasping, but I feel I am "doing something about it" when I swallow the vitamins. Maybe the placebo effect will work in my favor!

I have grown to the point where I feel myself to be of worth. I feel justified in taking up space. I am small, therefore I do not take up much. Perhaps someone some day will be glad that I did.

Living in the labyrinth can be lonely and frightening. Through this book and the support group, I have found company and courage to face the day.

AFTERWORD,
NOVEMBER 1993

It seems impossible that nearly two years have transpired since I first began this book. My "THC" (Therapist to Help Cope), Phyllis Dow, encouraged me to keep a daily journal chronicling my memory losses as therapy and later influenced me to submit it for publication.

I never expected a publisher to buy it. I didn't believe the world was ready for An Alzheimer's Who Talks—much less An Alzheimer's Who Talks Back! Even after a publisher finally bought it, my aspirations were small. I expected this book to be read only within the Alzheimer's community. The warm and enthusiastic response from the general public both here and abroad, as well as from the Alzheimer's community, has staggered me. I am profoundly moved.

With immense pride, I announce that the Early (Younger) Onset Patient Support Groups I initiated under the sponsorship of the Alzheimer's Association have spread across our nation and have helped many people affected by this disease.

I traveled by invitation to the 1992 Annual Meeting of the National Alzheimer's Association to address the representatives of chapters from all over the United States. My trip was chaperoned by one of our local board directors, Mary Ellen Ort-Marvin, and accompanied (as always!) by Richard Badessa, Ph.D., professor emeritus and a fellow traveler on our bridge of missing planks. Dear Richard, once converted to my way of thinking, has been my constant champion and has stood beside me throughout all my endeavors, with faith in me when I had none. Together, we stressed to the chapter representatives the importance of bonding with and relating to others like ourselves.

No matter how caring our caregivers may be, they cannot possibly imagine our grief as we attempt to cope with the trauma of our diagnosis. It takes "someone like me" to truly understand how I feel, what I think, and why. We share moral support and an esprit de corps such as the Marine Corps only dreams about. We trade experiences, solace, and enjoy the healing balm of shared laughter.

Laughter affords the same venting release as a scream . . . but is much more socially acceptable.

As groups we also stay updated on the most recent research, and some of our groups are actively participating in research projects. We feel that by doing so we are taking an active role in solving this dilemma. If advancements by the medical community are too late for some of us, we theorize, then we still have bettered the lot of those who come after us.

My pride in this accomplishment is such that I cannot express it in words . . . and I can be outspoken, but not by many.

I chafe, however, at the reluctance of some parts of the medical community to accept the good works those of us with Alzheimer's are performing, for and by ourselves. One doctor advised me he had never before spoken with an AD patient with such "insight." "Never!" he exclaimed. I invited him to attend one of our group meetings and promised to introduce him to at least eleven others.

This attitude bothers all of us who receive an Alzheimer's diagnosis. By struggling to maintain a plateau through mental stimulation exercises (this manuscript was one), we are upsetting the medical applecart. If we succeed, our very success confuses the heck out of the medical professionals who would be much more comfortable if we resigned ourselves to rapid deterioration, relinquished our tenuous hold on cognitive ability, and sank to the state of the severely devastated. Then, we realize, we would fit the "mold." Then we would not confuse the "unaffected experts" by proclaiming ourselves "affected experts."

As nuclear medicine's diagnostic capabilities constantly improve, more of us will be diagnosed earlier in the disease. We take small comfort in the fact that our numbers are increasing daily; however, as more of us boldly step forth and shoulder our own yokes, the general public and even the medical professionals will gradually become accustomed to our "insight" and willingness to participate in our own destinies.

Since this book was written, I am gratefully pleased to announce that my family is finally catching up with "What's wrong with Mom, anyway?" My children champion my efforts and proclaim their pride in my reluctance to take this neuro-glitch-from-hell sitting down. My husband has even come around, more slowly than the children, but progress has been made. While he openly states he still dreams of awaking someday to find this has all been a horrible nightmare, he is facing the reality of our situation. When we married, he did not know that "for better or worse" included Alzheimer's Disease . . . but then, neither did I.

He not only gives me more patience and understanding then he did initially, he grants me full rein to push my envelope as far as I can, without restraint. His only request is that he be permitted to avoid any and all limelight as a result of my illness, books, or being an "Affected Advocate" for more research funds, beneficial legislation on both national and state levels, and my efforts within my support group. He has become accustomed to emergency phone calls from a newly diagnosed and distraught member of our "club." He is aware that our "club" is quite exclusive . . . so much so, no one wants to be in it.

The biggest step my husband made was when he volunteered to master my little word processor to aid me when, or if, I lose the ability to operate my best means of communication with the outside world. So jealous am I of my little word processor friend that at first I only let my husband practice on an old broken-down one we owned. Nothing must happen to "my" friend, the word processor. It acts as my memory. It spells for me. It even corrects my grammar . . . sometimes. It never tells me to speak faster or to slow down. It permits me time to think. It permits me corrections.

As I read over this book, taking the reader from my first symptoms through diagnosis and my denial, I realize how far I have come psychologically, if not intellectually. *Living in the Labyrinth* was written in a state of grief such as I'd never experienced, and it jumps out at me as I read back over the pages. However, life was meant to be lived, not endured. And live it I shall.

With my husband's dogged skills at the word processor, I've continued to keep a journal. It is written with an eye towards coping, and when I reread it I am reminded that, even with Alzheimer's, life can be fun . . . if you know how to play it.

All my news is not happy, however. I have sustained some additional losses, most noticeably in the frontal lobe area. As a result, I am more emotional, greatly impulsive; rumor has it I sometimes display a lack of judgment, and my "oil factories" (olfactory senses) really create havoc. I spent three days searching my home for the cause of the unpleasant odor of urine. More specifically, cat urine. Not owning a cat, I watched my dear little terrier with suspicion and repeatedly emptied the vacuum cleaner bag, all to no avail. Finally, my husband advised me that there was no such offensive odor; it was my "oil factories" again.

Not all of these new losses and developments are unpleasant, however. I can sometimes enjoy the sweet fragrance of night-blooming jasmine, when no one else can. It is my own private and enjoyable sensation.

I am aware (having so much "insight," y'know) that this means the disease is, indeed, progressing within me. I can handle it, however.

Have you ever experienced and enjoyed the fragrance of night-blooming jasmine?

AFTERWORD,
NOVEMBER 1994

Dear Reader,

This addition to *Living In The Labyrinth* is written as a
further update on the status of myself as an AD
patient and of the growth of the nationwide network
of Early Onset Support Groups which I spearheaded
in 1992. It will also shed a lot of light on what hap-
pens when the slower moving Alzheimer patient is
thrust into the fast lane of media attention and the
publishing world.

This is an accounting which must be presented, lest
anyone mistakenly believe that I differ from other
patients who constantly fear the very real possibility
of becoming "inappropriate" in the eyes of the unaffected. That fear grips me every time I step up to a
podium or attempt to appear relaxed before television cameras.

Nor must the reader be of the mistaken opinion that

127

because I have gone public, said public cuts me any slack. At times I have felt like the bait in a shark pool, defenseless against those who would take a bite of me.

If I am to list the numerous positives gained by the affected population and their families through a modicum of public attention, it would be a cop-out not to list the negatives also.

And I have never been accused of being a "cop-out."

I am frequently asked in interviews what one word of advice I'd like to give to my fellow AD patients. I have pondered that in the past, and have occasionally come up with a word or two of wisdom. Now, however, I feel I have this thing in perspective, and the best advice I could give an Alzheimer patient is, "Don't write a book!"

Were it not for my stubbornness and desperation to campaign for patients' rights and assistance, I'd have gulped down a large dose of hemlock early in this effort. It is the kind, gracious concern of some unaffected and the enthusiasm and gratitude of the affected that has kept me going.

The general public is ready to listen, and the medical professionals even cast a jaundiced eye of interest at a book written by someone affected. Fellow patients are enthusiastic, praise me for my advocacy efforts and clamor for more; my mail and phone have both been on overload for a long while.

Not all of my experiences have been bad, of course. Delacorte has been as much of a lifesaver as an author could ever dream of, and I am grateful to them for their patience and consideration. The entire staff has treated me with *dignity and compassion*. This positive attitude is all the more outstanding when held up against the attitudes of others.

However, I would like to emphasize that no AD patient should enter into contracts of any sort without professional advice. I discovered late that just because an enterprise specializes in either products or services for Alzheimer's affected families, this specialization does not mean they differ from anyone else who might see a way to make a buck from another's diminished capacities. I encountered this lack of empathy and/or conscience when enterprising individuals who did not even know what Alzheimer's Disease was asked me to endorse "treatments" or "cures." (I declined.)

So when interest arose from film companies wanting to produce a television movie of my Life Story, I thought: Red flag! Red flag!

My husband ran for cover. My children ran to investigate a name change. I ran for representation by an agent. This time, I vowed, I had to have someone on my side.

As I write this, I believe the count is now up to three agencies involved (including one for the film studio) in the acquisition of film rights to My Life. It seems that everyone else required representation to combat the Alzheimer Woman who was finally getting Smart.

The media attention has been overwhelming. Newspapers ran articles about the Alzheimer Wannabe-Author from the little suburb outside Orlando. National magazines covered me, one spending four days with me (two for the journalist, and later, two for the photographer), and local, national, and even international television and radio interviews were conducted.

One day I spoke for five minutes on the telephone with a person I thought was conducting a scheduled Canadian live radio interview before discovering I was speaking with one of the California film producers.

A national television newsmagazine was the most heinous experience of my public exposure. They came into my little home for a scheduled two or three days of filming which somehow expanded to a total of twenty wretched days, all for a fifteen minute airing.

I received, it must be noted, no money for any of this. I was gritting my teeth and doing it for The Cause. They were doing it for The Buck . . . and The Ratings.

The production crew agreed quickly—too quickly, I now know—to everything I asked for in the manner of protection from harm and preservation of dignity, not only for myself and my family, but also for a dear friend and fellow patient, Richard Badessa, Ph.D., who gallantly stood by my side throughout all my efforts. I felt quite betrayed when the segment aired. Incidents and comments we thought were off the record were there for all to see. My fears of my own inappropriate behavior were realized in shots of me stammering and crying as a result of the stress of the filming. I let the producer know just how I felt:

Dear apologetic Mr. Producer Man,

Thank you for your many admissions to having done

me wrong.

Glad you had time to enjoy Bermuda. Nothing like sea breezes to clear cobwebs from the mind. And the eyes of jaundiced producer-types who use Ugly Old Woman lenses.

Since my debut:

1. My daughter phoned asking what had "they" done to me as she had just seen me the week before and I didn't look like that.

2. Old school friend (Kurt Fuller in book) phoned from NY to ask for reaffirmation that "we aren't really seventy years old, are we, Diane?"

3. Dell reps did not recognize me when they came to La Guardia to pick me up. (I looked younger than they'd expected. They recognized my husband or would have walked past me.)

4. In public, people rush up to me to say I certainly look much younger and better than they had seen on "that TV show" the other night. "Which one did you see?" I ask, knowing already.

5. A member of the support group called to say now did I understand why they won't ever go public as I have.

6. Two aunts phoned to say I looked older than my mother did when she died, while another phoned to say whatever I had done between your show and *Sonya Live*, keep it up; I had improved A LOT!

7. I've had correspondence and calls from people wanting to sell me lotsa vitamin, mineral, and herbal cures; one told me to become Born Again while there was still time.

A man said he noticed from the photographs and my appearance on the show that I must be ailing not from Alzheimer's but from "that disease that ages a person quickly and prematurely."

Another sent a pendulum to check my electromagnetic field.

A woman offered to come live w/us for $2,000–$3,000 per month to deoxygenize me.

Another said to just rub my ears and my memory will improve . . . actually, I think it was the bone in front of or behind my ears, can't really remember . . .

MANY have referred to my husband as a "jerk off," "dud," and (expletive deleted), adding they hope I am getting it on with Richard. . . .

And . . . how do I get my teeth so white?

I reply that I'll take their advisement under consideration . . . and I use Crest.

Tell your expectant wife I send my best and NOT to let you into the delivery room with camera crew. That is not ever a woman's best angle.

Forget Me Never,
/S/ Diana Friel McGowin

Throughout all of the above, I was definitely out of my depth, but Fate itself got my revenge. During one beach shot when the cameraman and soundman were perched in the backseat of my little convertible, the producer called to me to lower the top. I obliged, and the power top caught both men and their equipment, nearly scalping the cameraman and stopping the taping for a while due to snared equipment.

Mr. Producer Man instructed me to "get rid" of two parrots in my living room for a day's shoot. I put one bird outside in the aviary, and perched the other one inside the bathroom shower. Later, the producer needed to relieve himself and entered the bathroom. Just at the worst possible moment, my little parrot gave a wolf whistle, called out a cheery "Hello," and the producer nearly wet down my bathroom walls.

During the last day of their outdoor filming, prehurricane gales and rain torrents flooded their expensive equipment.

The cameraman was mugged in our local airport.

As a result of the media attention, people began recognizing me on the street. They always meant well, but it was disconcerting, particularly for an Alzheimer patient, to be approached by so many smiling strangers. We are confronted in our daily lives by acquaintances whom we no longer recognize, and the world suddenly became populated with these individuals.

One lady observed me being escorted by my son through the airport in Washington, D.C. She followed me through the airport without either my son or me noticing her, and waited until I stepped away from my son momentarily. She approached me swiftly then, and after first exclaiming her delight in meeting me, she smiled in compassion.

"I'm so sorry your husband is like he is," she said, referring to my husband's taciturn manner toward me as it had been revealed by the television newsmagazine. "But I'm glad you have your friend the professor," she added, still smiling.

A small group began gathering. I could no longer see the whereabouts of my escorting son, who was wondering how I could have disappeared so quickly in an international airport. A handsome young man in military uniform agreed with the compassionate lady and confided that he had been unable to get me out of his mind since the show had aired, worrying that my husband will not take care of me.

133

Dear God, I thought.

One week later, I received in the mail a copy of my book with a request for an autograph. The note was signed, "The lady who followed you in the airport."

Other national television interviews were not quite as hurtful nor demeaning as the one I described, but my nerves had begun to fail, and neither my doctors nor I could tell where frontal lobe involvement left off and sheer exhaustion began.

It all came to a climax following a speech at a prominent medical center.

In addition to the book publicity I had also been championing the cause of the Early Onset patient through speaking engagements under the auspices of the Alzheimer Association or various university medical centers and civic groups. Richard had cut back his schedule and was openly worried that I was flying in the face of the big enemy of the Alzheimer patient, stress, by not reducing my own activities. He warned me incessantly that I was sacrificing myself.

However, I felt driven. While the public interest was up, I wanted to keep driving home the message that Early Onsets do, indeed, exist, and we must be reckoned with.

I was invited to be the sole speaker for a fund-raiser at a major hospital's Alzheimer center. It was quite successful, and I met some very dedicated and caring professional caregivers. However, as I was being escorted to a car for my flight home, I suddenly collapsed.

It was as though I had been unplugged. I grabbed for a nearby building wall, discovered to my dismay it was polished marble, could not grasp it, and slid like a rag doll down the smooth surface.

During the embarrassing hubbub which ensued, as my escort had a panic attack and others watched in dismay, I insisted that I be taken to the airport for my return flight. Why? Because early the next morning I had another speech to give, and then a Canadian radio phone interview.

They held the plane up, while I, carrying my high heels in my arms, was escorted aboard by the pilot. Again, not one of my better moments.

It was time for another battery of neuropsych tests. I had been taking an anti-inflammatory medication recently discovered to be beneficial to AD patients because it reduces inflammation in the brain. I was experiencing pronounced improvement in the fluidity of my speech, some memory enhancement, and generally, a higher level of functioning, and I joyfully announced this to my neurologist. Still, he scheduled the dreaded, exhausting battery of tests.

"You mean you won't just take my word for it?" I asked.

"Nope. Take the tests, Diane."

The tests indicate I am still basically in a holding pattern, on a "plateau," that favorite of Alzheimer buzzwords. Still being on a plateau is significant to me because it supports what I have, in my "affected expert" state, maintained all along, and what recently some "unaffected experts" (medical professionals) are now touting too. Alzheimer's Disease is probably a *family* of neurological diseases. At one time cancer was simply cancer, but now we know that there are many types and varieties of cancer, requiring a variety of both diagnostic and treatment procedures. This family theory is the only plausible explanation as to why some AD patients decline with vicious rapidity, while others who receive the identical lab, clinical, and neuropsych test results remain on plateaus of precarious safety for indefinite periods of time.

I intend to maintain the longest plateau on record.

During one ignominious talk show interview, I received a phone call from a caregiver who could barely disguise her resentment of the fact that I (and others within my support group) have successfully maintained a plateau with no noticeable deterioration, while her own family patient had not. I weep inside for this woman, as well as her patient. But I also feel sharply a hurt, a bewilderment that instead of viewing my plateau as encouragement, a teeny ray of light in a darkening void, someone would resent me for still surviving.

I will not be reduced to apologizing for still being here giving this disease hell . . . but sometimes I truly am greatly tempted to do just that.

I have learned another lesson from this incident (and they say AD patients cannot learn!). I have learned that when you stand up to be counted, you make a dandy target.

Traveling to promote advocacy efforts on behalf of Alzheimer patients has presented problems, but has not been impossible. Any scheduling of trips must be made with an eye toward making sure the patient does not become either confused or exhausted. The patient must be escorted from pillar to post. Rest time must be incorporated into the schedule, as the sheer effort of focusing can be an immeasurable drain upon the AD patient. It is by "focusing," or channeling our energies into one tight circumference of attention, that we patients are able to "pass," or perform satisfactorily. We still have much to contribute, but must be granted our individual requirements for successfully contributing.

When Richard Badessa and I first traveled to Chicago in 1992 to address the national annual meeting of the Alzheimer's Association, we were properly chaperoned and escorted by a member of the Greater Orlando Alzheimer Board of Directors. Our escort, a young woman the age of my daughter, took her assignment very seriously, yet did not let her professionalism dim the experience of two Alzheimer patients who were the first on record ever to address the annual meeting of the national association. The exhilaration we felt as we successfully performed our duties on this trip was shared by all the professional representatives of chapters across the United States.

Early Onset Patient Support Groups are spreading like a wildfire across our nation. If they put anything on my epitaph, I want it to be that I began that movement; I am proudest of that and it is my benchmark. By forming support groups, we patients can take the reins of our life up in our own hands again, give one another solace and cheer, enjoy sustenance, and receive the determination to endure rather than simply give up and fade away, or, even worse, to prematurely "terminate," our not-so-cleverly-disguised word for suicide.

Due to both the acceptance of my book and the wide gamut of media attention it has received, patients have the privilege of communicating for the first time with others like themselves. My phone calls and correspondence with other Early Onset patients and their families have stretched from South Africa to the United Kingdom, from Australia to Nova Scotia, and I have as many Canadian "fellow travelers" as I have across the United States.

The book is now being accepted in Asian and Scandinavian countries, so we patients and others involved in Alzheimer advocacy can only expect our cause to continue to be championed around the world.

Nothing will slow us down, now that we are moving!

Alzheimer's Disease in all of its many forms plays no ethnic favorite. It is prevalent in Southwest Africa as well as in West Palm Beach.

And all of us ask the same two questions: First, we admit to a shallow, murmured, "Why me?" . . . and then the more strident, outraged scream, "Why no cure?"

I have networked with these many other patients via long distance, and our sharing by letters, audiotapes, videotapes, and telephone (whatever and whichever method we are capable of) means a great deal to each of us. I have found that, with rare exception, once a patient has a rapport with and the moral support of another, humor surfaces in finite degree, and sometimes can become the person's best persona.

That is why I still face the media, warts and all. I am learning to use the User. Without the media attention, we would not have discovered there are so many of us and had the benefit of joining hands around the globe. Without the media attention, professional caregivers would not now be reevaluating their individual attitudes toward their incognizant charges, people who are unfortunate to be just a bit further down the road than those of us who are still vocal.

Each time I am contacted by a "reformed" professional caregiver, I give a silent prayer of thanks. I may fall under that person's care someday.

I am often asked if I fear the ogre of Death connected with this terminal illness. I have never spoken with a patient who dwells on the terminal aspect of this neurological disease. We are much too concerned, and desperately so, with what lies between where we are today and the end. It is not the end which occupies our nightmares and daytime panics and causes a fear as gripping as a cold hand within our chests. It is how we reach that end.

We devote our time, attention, and energies to the road we are on, not the destination.

A major medical center released a medical report in 1993 wherein it was announced that the smile is usually the last to go. I don't believe that is an accident. I do believe it is significant.

When I look at my initial patient support group, now numbering more than twenty, and the many patients with whom I have networked across the

139

country, the past year presents a sobering, but still encouraging, picture.

Four have fallen from their tenuous individual plateaus into further deterioration and can no longer communicate with us well.

One of our founding group members died.

The rest of us remain, clinging to our plateaus.

We remain, we endure, we continue to fight for our rights, our dignity, and to spur researchers on toward a treatment of this disease with which we have been branded.

We feel like the living dinosaurs must have felt as they watched the Ice Age approach.

I am reminded of a clever patient's response when advised by his physician that while there are a few experimental drugs being researched, there is no cure for Alzheimer's Disease.

The patient responded, "There is no cure for premature ejaculation, either, but I understand it is coming fast."

Smile with us, my friend, smile with us.

Smile, and understand.

To you, you are holding a book in your hands. To us, you are holding our lives.

Forget Me Never,

DIANA FRIEL MCGOWIN

GLOSSARY

Alzheimer's Disease

A puzzling form of dementia seen in people as young as 28 years of age, but most often encountered later in life. The exact cause is not yet known but extensive research is being conducted. At present the only certain diagnosis is through autopsy of the brain tissue after death. However, a probable diagnosis can be determined on the living patient by scanning procedures such as the MRI and SPECT. Many neurologists are hesitant to base a firm diagnosis on these relatively new diagnostic tools, however. It is believed that as nuclear medicine improves and continues to develop finer diagnostic techniques, there will be an earlier diagnosis, and subsequently a treatment, for Alzheimer's.

Chemical Profile

A laboratory test of the blood to determine the ratio of various chemical compounds within the system. Frequently administered in conjunction with other blood tests.

CT Scan (Neurological)

The patient is injected with a radioisotope dye

through the vein of one arm, after which technicians conduct an x-ray of the brain and surrounding fluids.

Dementias

Neurological disorders symptomized by loss of capacity.

Early-Diagnosed

A term which means that the disease has been diagnosed early in its course. The term can apply equally to early-onset patients or individuals who first suffered symptoms at an elderly age.

Early-Onset

This term applies to those individuals diagnosed between the ages of 28 and 62.

EEG (Electroencephalogram)

A non-invasive diagnostic procedure in which the patient lies in a darkened room while electrodes are placed at strategic points of the head, and held in place by use of a putty. This gives a reading of electric impulses within the brain.

Hereditary Factor

Some of the premature dementias are due to an inherited factor.

Lumbar Puncture (Spinal Tap)

Fluid is removed from the patient's lower spine and analyzed for causative agents which would denote a usually treatable neurological/chemical dysfunction.

MRI
(Magnetic Resonance Imaging, Neurological)

A neurological scan of the brain which permits an in-depth view of all brain tissue, both white and grey matter. The procedure produces a film which illustrates "slices" of the brain for close examination and review by the neurologist.

Multi-Infarct Dementia

A dementia whereby the patient suffers multiple "infarcts" or breakdowns of the vascular system within the brain, such as both minor and major strokes.

SPECT Brain Scan

A brain scan which can detect the presence of isotopes which are indicative of Alzheimer's disease.

TIA
(Transient Ischemic Attack or Transient Ischemic Episode)

A minor stroke, sometimes occuring due to hypertension, but not necessarily related to high blood pressure. Sufficient numbers of TIAs can result in "multi-infarct" (multiple infarcations)— areas where the damaged blood supply of the brain no longer feeds that particular area, and thereby renders the affected tissue incapable of performing its neurological task.

❦

Medical Notes by Michael Mullan, M.D.

Living in the Labyrinth is a chronicle of one woman's experience of the early stages of a disorder known to clinicians as dementia. As physicians, relatives, and friends, we recognize the syndrome of dementia by the progressive loss of memory, of other intellectual capacities, and of personality. These clinical features of Alzheimer's Disease (AD) and other dementias arise as a result of the degeneration and death of brain cells. Dementia in late life is common, affecting an estimated four million Americans, but is uncommon at the age that Diane McGowin first began to experience symptoms. Of the causes of dementia, AD is the commonest, followed by multi-infarct dementia (MID), which is due to vascular disease, cardiac disease, and/or hypertension. These risk factors for developing MID are well-known, but for the majority of cases of AD neither the causes nor effective treatments are known. Implicit in the diagnosis of AD are the ideas that there is no underlying other cause and that there will generally be steady decline.

This helps us classify the disease, but it does not help us to explain it; the cause of the Alzheimer's degenerative brain damage is unknown in all but a relatively small number of cases.

Dementia most commonly afflicts the elderly and does so at a time in their lives when they most need their mental faculties to deal with the challenges of retirement. Dementia strikes the young much less frequently, but the consequences are generally catastrophic for the victim and the family. Occupation, relationships, and mental health bear the brunt of the onslaught of deterioration as the ability to think, reason, and communicate declines. In the young age group, the impact in these areas of life is often dramatic. Premature retirement, strained marriages, or divorce, depression, and anxiety are common accompaniments. As described here, these areas became problems for Diane, but perhaps her response to them is unusual in that she is able to fully appreciate what is happening to her and doggedly refuses to be overwhelmed.

The first signs of AD, such as forgetting shopping lists or recent visitors, are common symptoms often noticed by family members. Disorientation with respect to time, place, and person is another early feature. In her chapter "Unplanned Journey," Diane describes disorientation regarding place after a period of confusion, dizziness, and falling (syncope) as well as slurred speech, which are characteristic of transient ischaemic attacks (TIAs). TIAs, which are due to a fleeting loss of blood supply to the brain, are quite commonly related to multi-infarct dementia and not to Alzheimer's Disease. Later, in "Initial Testing," Diane describes her inability to recognize a close relative. This is one of a variety of losses of knowledge (agnosia) that afflicts the dementing patient. Again, in Alzheimer's Disease this is not often a reversible phenomenon. Usually, as the dementing process progresses, there is a loss of the ability to use language in an appropriate way and an inability to understand the spoken and written word. This loss of ability to communicate naturally results in frustration that may be expressed as verbal or physical aggression. Later, in Alzheimer's Disease there is loss of the function of coordinated movement, and the patient becomes progressively bed bound. At this stage, fits (seizures), strokes, and Parkinson-like movements are common. Death usually occurs as a complication of immobility and is often partly a relief for caregivers, as by this stage the person they once knew is frequently not recognizable. The duration of this whole process in Alzheimer's Disease is approximately eight years, although there is great variation from one patient to the next.

Most commonly in the early stages of dementia (especially Alzheimer's), insight is mercifully lost and the victim drifts without self-awareness into the depths of the illness. Other sufferers have a disorder that takes a different course with retained self-knowledge. Diane McGowin clearly falls into this latter group and with alarming insight has transcribed her understanding of her predicament, giving us a vivid description of life with a disorder that erodes intellect and personality. As readers, we are taken through the stages of awareness of the early symptoms, the diagnostic process, and the impact of the cognitive problems on her everyday life.

The diagnosis of Alzheimer's Disease is made by excluding other causes of dementia. There is currently no known effective treatment for the disease,

147

so the identification of other causes of dementia is key, because many of them have identifiable and treatable causes. Multi-infarct dementia, for instance, is associated with a variety of factors that can be influenced, such as atherosclerosis, hypertension, and heart disease. The control and management of these underlying disorders can potentially halt the progression of multi-infarct dementia. Another common cause of dementia is alcohol, and a history or evidence of alcohol abuse is carefully sought during clinical assessment. Tumors, hormonal abnormalities, vitamin deficiencies, and many other processes can lead to dementia, but these are much rarer than dementia caused by the Alzheimer's process.

No single current test unequivocally determines the diagnosis; rather, tests are used as diagnostic aids to confirm good clinical judgment. A good clinical history of all other medical conditions is paramount, and a general examination is usually performed. The clinical assessment of dementia begins with a detailed history of the development of the disease from the patient (which is often unreliable), relative, or caregiver, or usually all of these. Medical and nursing notes help to date the appearance of the first signs and symptoms, which are most commonly loss of memory for recently acquired information and events. (My most memorable example of this is of a patient who forgot to switch off her gas cooker and started a fire in her home, which fortunately was extinguished by water pouring through the ceiling from a neglected tap in her bath). Details of the mood and personality changes are important—some cases of severe depression masquerade as dementia, but depression and anxiety are also (not surprisingly) common accompaniments of the early stages of intellectual decline. Bedside tests of memory orientation, attention, and concentration are commonly administered by physicians to give them a feel for any serious intellectual problems, but detailed testing by a psychologist is sometimes required, especially in the early stages. A series of routine blood tests help to exclude dementia due to rarer conditions. EEGs and scans are generally used to confirm the impression gained during interview. CT or MRI scans are usually more than sufficient to confirm a diagnosis of dementia and may give additional information on localization of degeneration of brain tissue and therefore some important clues to the cause. For instance, Alzheimer's Disease may begin in one area of the brain and characteristically spread throughout the cortical (outermost) areas of the brain. MID, by contrast, may have a very localized pattern in these scans. The diagnosis of Alzheimer's is made in accordance with nationally determined criteria. In deference to the difficulties of diagnosis and the essential pathological nature of the diagnosis, three categories are recognized: possible, probable, and definite Alzheimer's. A diagnosis of definite Alzheimer's can only be made at autopsy; experienced clinicians, however, will accurately diagnose Alzheimer's with up to 95 percent accuracy using the above approach.

Many of the difficulties of the diagnostic process are highlighted in Diane's case. The not uncommon case of double diagnosis of MID *and* Alzheimer's is especially difficult to disentangle. A step-wise deterioration of mental abilities closely related to stroke-like episodes is the hallmark of MID. An insidious and slowly progressive dementing process unrelated to stroke episodes is more characteristic of AD. Nevertheless, despite these clinical guidelines, misdiagnosis of both AD and MID quite frequently occurs.

Clearly, we still need to find out much more about
the relationship and natural history of these common conditions. Fortunately, many first-class research institutes are addressing these issues, using
clinical experience as well as new scanning and psy-
chometric techniques to form the final diagnosis.

There is no proven drug treatment now available
that will halt the Alzheimer's process once it has
started. Some currently available research drugs may
ameliorate the symptoms in some cases. The efficacy
of such drugs is still being evaluated, but it is most
unlikely that they will reverse or halt the underlying
degenerative process. What then causes the brain
cells to die? This is the riddle of Alzheimer's to
which many international scientists are applying
themselves with the belief that finding the cause will
lead to the cure. One twist of the riddle which we are
coming to appreciate is that not all Alzheimer's is
caused by the same thing. My colleagues have identi-
fied clear genetic causes of the disease. Before I
discuss these findings and their implications in detail, it should be made clear that the proportion
of Alzheimer's cases caused by simple errors in genes
is very small and that the cause in the majority of
late-onset cases is still unknown.

Early-onset Alzheimer's cases have made a key contribution to our understanding of the disease. Familial early-onset cases are caused by genetic errors
transmitted from affected individuals to their children with 50 percent chance. The first and only
presently known cause of Alzheimer's was shown to
be a genetic error in a gene encoding a protein
called amyloid. Amyloid has long been known to
Alzheimer's researchers as the deposit which occurs
in the brains of all sufferers. What was not known

was whether amyloid deposition was a cause or a consequence of the disease. The discovery of genetic "spelling mistakes" in a gene unequivocally showed that amyloid was the sole cause in these rare early-onset familial cases. This finding places amyloid in the center of the search for the causes of all cases of the disease. Although the question of the role of amyloid remains to be answered in the case of late-onset disease, it is clear that the patients with early-onset disease who volunteered for the genetic research made a very significant contribution. Diane, who discovers that her mother too had suffered from early-onset intellectual decline ("Friends for All Seasons"), is an advocate of research and has volunteered to take part in early-onset genetic studies. By contributing in this way, victims of dementia and their families and friends learn more of the realities of these disorders (a two-edged sword) but make critical contributions to our understanding of these diseases. Ultimately, their participation leads directly to rational therapies for these disorders. This point is rarely made but may be the most important consequence of the genetic research. By inserting the mutations into cultured cells (or experimental animals), we can reproduce key early features of the disease process in the laboratory. One immediate implication for such test systems is that they can be used to rapidly screen for potentially therapeutic compounds. A recently discovered genetic mutation (causing Alzheimer's Disease) in Sweden is already allowing us to do exactly that. In cells the mutation causes the overproduction of amyloid. In the victims who inherit this mutation the whole gamut of clinical and neuropathological features are caused by this genetic defect in β-amyloid. A cultured neuronal cell with this mutation will begin to reproduce the whole disease process. This is the first system of many of its kind and is being used by a major drug company to screen for drugs that will prevent the early stages of the disease as mimicked in these cells.

Reading this rare personal account of cognitive loss, we are struck, not only by the emotional accompaniments—fear, shame, and anguish—but also by the good humor and sharp insights Diane brings to bear on her predicament. Despite these irrational processes, Diane maintains an earnest and rational commitment to research. She rightly believes that the understanding and treatment of the condition from which she suffers will come from meticulous application of the scientific method. This does not always move as quickly as we would like. There is no doubt that the voluntary entry into research studies by sufferers like Diane speeds this process.

Finally, it is worth noting that Diane's piercing insight into her mental state is uncharacteristic of AD—the faculty of self-awareness often being sacrificed early. Fortunately, it is the preservation of these mental capacities that make such a book possible. These variations in the clinical picture and the difficulties of diagnosis should turn our attention to support groups directed at AD and related disorders to ensure support for those individuals who do not easily fit the diagnostic picture but nevertheless need and deserve as much support as more easily recognizable cases receive.

Who else needs support? Well, undoubtedly the friends, relatives, and carers do. Witnessing the demise of a loved one is understandably difficult. The time from learning to understanding and accepting the diagnosis, the period of self-education, and the search for treatments are characteristic phases through which the caregivers pass. Support and well-informed counsel are essential to make these phases as healthy as possible. Perhaps this book will help them to understand the frustrations and anguish of the dementia victim, which is often only matched by their own. Many of the unspoken themes of dementia are illuminated by Diane. Changes in sexuality and domestic relationships—usually never discussed—are explicitly recorded by Diane. The provision of a receptive environment in which these delicate but profoundly human issues can be discussed is an important goal and will help us all to understand better this group of illnesses as research works to provide the much needed treatments.

Michael Mullan, M.D.,
University of South Florida,
April 1993.

Appendix 2

WARNING SYMPTOMS
FOR EARLY ONSET ALZHEIMER'S DISEASE

The early-onset patient is often still active in his or her career, family, social obligations, hobbies and religious persuasion when productivity is suddenly cut short. Some falter much more rapidly than others; some level off at a plateau where they remain for as many as 9 or10 years before sustaining further deterioration or perhaps dying of an unrelated cause. This appendix lists the most common symptoms. All symptoms do not apply to all patients, however.

If anyone reading this list recognises the warning signs, they should undergo a complete and thorough physical immediately. Many other treatable and curable ailments can cause symptoms similar to Alzheimer's disease.

Checklist

- Unusual confusion and short-term (recent) memory loss occurs, akin to a transient, innocuous blight. You may remember the information tomorrow, but not today, when it is needed.

- Becoming lost, even temporarily, in what should be familiar surroundings. Anyone can lose their house keys. If you have the keys but cannot find your house, you're in trouble.

- Losing your label system. Cannot recall the names of well-known people or even family members.

- Work efficiency spirals downward, causing

155

great anxiety, tension, depression. Everything seems to overwhelm you.

- Speech is usually fluent, but you may suddenly lose a key word in mid-sentence. You improvise by substituting another word which may not be appropriate.

- You have to carry notes around in order to perform the most routine duties or errands.

- You become secretive, hiding away evidence of your lapses of orientation or memory.

- You always seem to be looking for a lost item.

- Weight loss is sometimes experienced, as is insomnia.

- Sudden change in sexuality, libido. Usually this is an acceleration; however some male patients experience impotency.

- Spatial concept is sometimes affected; you experience awkward accidents or clumsiness.

- Your language may become saltier than in the past and you may dress or behave inappropriately in a momentary lapse of decorum. ❧

ᘐᓷ

ADVICE FOR CAREGIVERS

I have been deeply touched by the love and affection shown by my husband, family and friends in recent months. The most important care a loved one can give the patient is *consistent* demonstration of love and support. Not just a dutiful standing by with a "Gee whiz!" attitude; not aiding the patient in their denials; or debilitating them even further by confronting them with their losses. A sincere, comforting and reassuring presence is called for.

One would have to be divine to ascertain always when to be firm and when to be gentle, when to confront and when to remain silent, when the patient needs to be held and comforted and when to be left to sit alone in reverie. Since you are not divine, I recommend you pray for divine guidance. The patient is — all the time.

Following is a list of suggestions to make the lives of patient and caregiver easier.

- Even though it will not always be easy, try to give the patient boundless love, leisure and laughter. All kindnesses, large or small, are very much appreciated. As much as a thoughtless or angry word can injure, so can kindness, grace, and gentleness heal. Through the patient's own mushrooming insecurity, a greater sensitivity for others and an infinite gratitude develops.

- Whenever their burden exasperates or embarrasses you, try to comprehend (you are the cognizant one, remember) how great is their own humiliation as they travel their undeserved and unrequested road.

- Try to keep the patient interested in hobbies, supervising him, if necessary. Reading, even if the material is not always retained, should be continued until the patient reaches the point when the effort is entirely pointless. Audio books work well and are available from most libraries. While many patients experience a gradual loss of visual comprehension, auditory abilities falter more slowly.

- Once you have adjusted to your relative's condition, counseling with the family attorney can be very helpful. A Power of Attorney and Guardianship should be effected for the protection of the patient and family, alike. These legal documents are best drafted while the patient has some understanding of their purpose and while he can still participate in their preparation.

- Keep a good, clear, recent photograph of the patient on hand. Should he become lost or wander away from home, this photo can be circulated to help locate him.

- The patient should not travel by bus or train without an escort. Buses and trains make numerous stops and a confused patient may wrongfully disembark. Airplane travel is possible, but you must book a 'non-stop' flight.

Booking a 'non-change' flight is not enough, as the patient may become confused by the stop and exit the aircraft. It **must** be non-stop.
Make sure that the patient carries a note giving his name, destination and a telephone number. Escort him to the gate, and make solid arrangements to have him met on arrival. Inform the airline attendants of the patient's condition, and give them a recent photograph.
Attendants are trained to assist handicapped passengers and to keep a watchful eye on them. In the later stages the patient must always be accompanied by a caregiver when traveling.

- It is essential that the patient and family try their utmost to keep a healthy sense of humor alive. There are some opprobious situations which will befall you and your only salvation will be the grace of laughter. It provides the same venting release as a scream, but is much more socially acceptable.

- Check into the availability of support groups for you, the caregiver, and also for the patient. Many support groups exist for caregivers, guiding them through each phase of the disease and providing them with moral support. Unfortunately, there are fewer support groups for patients, even though the need to share fears and give and receive moral support is as great, if not more so. If you can't find a support group in your locale, then start one. I did, and I'm the patient. ☜☞

159

USEFUL ADDRESSES

Alzheimer's Association
919 North Michigan Ave., Suite 1000
Chicago IL 60611-1676
1-800-272-3900

*This organization provides literature, moral support and
counseling resources to families and caregivers.*

Alzheimer's Disease Education & Referral Center
P.O. Box 8250, Silver Springs MD 20907-8250
301-495-3311

Alzheimer's Disease Society of Canada
491 Lawrence Ave. West, #501,
Toronto, Ontario, Canada M5M1C7

Society for the Right to Die
250 West 57th Street, New York NY 10107
212-246-6973

*This non-profit organization provides Living Wills and
Durable Powers of Attorney for Health Care. It gives advice
on the laws regarding patients' rights in particular medical
situations and publishes a member newsletter.
Annual membership is $15.*

*If you would like to contact the author and find out more
about her early-onset support group, her address is:*

Diane Friel McGowin
P.O. Box 585072, Orlando FL 32858-5072

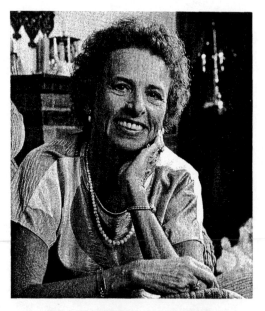

DIANA FRIEL McGOWIN
founded the early-onset support group
in her hometown of Orlando, Florida,
following her diagnosis in 1991.
With her condition stabilized, she
remains active in the local Alzheimer's
Association and networks with
other victims.